Vicci Bentley has specialized in health, beauty and lifestyle journalism for over twenty-five years. Her articles have appeared in magazines including *Cosmopolitan*, *Woman's Journal* and *Marie Claire*. She is currently Beauty Director of *Good Housekeeping*.

GW00691731

LOSE TEN YEARS IN TEN MINUTES A DAY

VICCI BENTLEY

ORION

An Orion Paperback
First published in Great Britain in 2001 by
Orion Books Ltd,
Orion House, 5 Upper St Martin's Lane,
London WC2H 9EA

Copyright © 2001 Vicci Bentley
Illustrations copyright © 2001 Ceri Staziker

The right of Vicci Bentley to be identified as the author of
this work has been asserted by her in accordance with the
Copyright, Designs and Patents Act 1988.

All rights reserved. No part of this publication may be
reproduced, stored in a retrieval system, or transmitted, in
any form or by any means, electronic, mechanical,
photocopying, recording or otherwise, without the prior
permission of the copyright owner.

A CIP catalogue record for this book
is available from the British Library.

ISBN: 0 75281 731 0

Printed and bound in Great Britain by
The Guernsey Press Co. Ltd, Guernsey, C.I.

CONTENTS

CHAPTER 1

Motivation
Yes, you can look younger in minutes

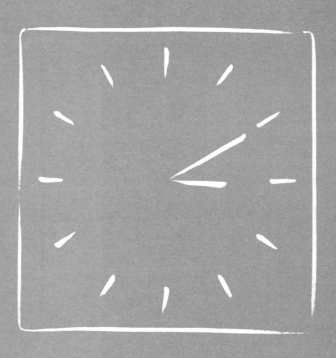

The secret of looking younger is refusing to look older – and there's a lot out there that helps. Cosmetics help brighten our outlook and smooth the impact of lines. Diet and exercise keep body and soul in tune, helping us to stay fit and looking younger, longer. What's the motivating factor that keeps us glowing on? Attitude. We do it because we can. And the best news of all? It gets better by the minute.

'Anti-ageing' was the buzzword of 1990s beauty culture. Now we're into the new millennium, 'stay fit' and 'stay young' are familiar lifestyle mantras. There's never been a better time to reach prime time. Women aged 35 and over account for the fastest growing sector of global population. Market researchers Mintel predict that by the year 2003, these 'baby boomers' will account for 40% of UK citizens with a vested interest in maximizing their vitality.

But what does anti-ageing really mean? Sheer demand already means that there is a bewildering choice of sophisticated beauty products on the market. No wonder we're dazed and confused! But let's get this straight: looking younger isn't about chasing idealistic claims and promises offered by slick, costly cosmetics.

The best practical anti-ageing advice is to make an investment in the future of your good looks and wellbeing. Outwardly, you can prevent the acceleration of the more obvious age giveaways, like lines and wrinkles. Inwardly, you can practise sound health strategies, such as

> *Inner vitality knocks years off your image*

nutrition, exercise and stress-beating relaxation that will offset the many age-related diseases that make us old before our time. Inner vitality knocks years off your image – when you feel good, you look fabulous. And there's proof.

A few years ago, a survey of over 6000 women carried out by the American magazine *New Woman* revealed that younger women fear ageing most, dreading loss of vitality, life choices and sexual desirability. Older women, however, experience middle and old age as a time of opportunity, when they can stop caring so much about beauty and what others think and focus instead on what makes them happy. Most encouragingly, many older women reported that they were more interested in sex than ever before – and about half of those interviewed had a younger lover.

Another US study, at the Wellesley Centre for Research on Women, compared women aged 35 to 55 and also discovered that the middle years have it going for them. Instead of the decline in mental health they had expected, researchers found that most women looked forward to renewed self-worth and greater confidence – in short, a beautiful new lease of life. Ageing expert Dr John Rowe at Mount Sinai Hospital and School of Medicine in New York agrees: the older you get, the more you feel in control of your life, he says. And that's the key to staying happy and healthy.

According to the results of a recent British survey carried out by Dr Ian Stuart Hamilton of Worcester College and commissioned by the skincare company RoC, not only did the vast majority of the 322 women interviewed believe a positive attitude to be the key to staying young,

> *We can control the way we age*

> ## Confidence is a woman's most powerfully sexy ally

they were adamant that we can control the way we age. 98 per cent thought that light exercise keeps the body young and lively, and 76 per cent said beauty products help control outward signs of ageing. Encouragingly, only 15 per cent believed cosmetic surgery to be the most effective anti-ageing treatment!

Dr Hamilton feels his survey shows a real change in the way women regard ageing. 'This positive approach to getting older and the belief that age is a state of mind demonstrate that women are feeling more in control of how they are perceived within society,' he says. 'The focus now is on how women feel inside. They are no longer slaves to the physical ageing process but can be the age they want to be.'

Confidence is a woman's most powerfully sexy ally – and if age brings more of it, we should feel more beautiful by the year. Perhaps this is why the fashion and beauty industry finally prizes its older icons as sassy role models. Achingly beautiful at 48, Isabella Rossellini inspires us to experiment with her Manifesto makeup range. 1970s icon, supermodel Karen Graham, recently came back from retirement to front Estée Lauder's Resilience Lift, a firming formula for 40+ skin. With thirty years of modelling behind her, Dayle Haddon is the face of l'Oréal's Plenitude Révitalift skincare range. 'I prefer to focus on all I have gained over the years, rather than dwell on what I may have lost in beauty terms,' she says. 'The key to looking good is feeling good and for me that means exercise, good quality relaxation, nutrition and serious skincare, which includes wearing a sunscreen even on a cloudy day.'

In the UK, model Harriet Close finds herself in increasing demand at 48. She also runs a model agency specializing in women over 30 – one of her newest recruits is in her 70s! 'As little as five years ago, girls would retire at around 30. Now their careers are being revitalized,' she says. Close sees the burgeoning anti-ageing market as a key reason for her girls' popularity. 'We're all living longer and keen to take care of ourselves. But we don't want to see 16-year-olds advertising our wrinkle creams. We need faces we can relate to.'

The wiser we get, the easier it is to motivate ourselves into feeling and looking great, whatever our age. Just listen to these 'veterans' of the anti-ageing game.

'Turning 30 doesn't threaten me. At 25, you've only got everyone else's word that wrinkles happen and your boobs start to drop. You can't appreciate what they're talking about because you think they still look great. Older women are so very much more attractive – everything they do is more confident, sophisticated and classy. Yasmin Le Bon looks fantastic, even after three kids. Sharon Stone has huge amounts of sex appeal. If that's what I have to look forward to, why worry?' Charlotte, 29, estate agent.

'People behave as though 30 is the end of their life. But this is the decade when I'm getting my act together, developing my character and moving in the direction I really want to. I'm so much more confident now and happier with the way I look. I wouldn't go back for anything – not even to 25.' Miranda, 32, complementary medicine practitioner.

'Life really can begin at 40. You do develop far more self-confidence. I used to constantly seek approval, but in the last two years I've discovered I no longer need sanction from others. I make my own decisions about how I look and I'm much more spontaneous and experimental in the way I dress. Healthwise, these are my insurance years – I'm determined to stay strong and fit for as long as I possibly can.' Pamela, 43, banker.

'I don't remember when I first noticed my wrinkles, it happened so gradually. But I certainly didn't panic. I cleanse and moisturize well, and protect myself against UV. I wear a lot less makeup now, because it's fashionable to look more natural. I've always worked hard to make myself presentable and boost my self-esteem. When I was younger, I tried to hide what I was feeling inside, but I'm so much more confident and happy where I am now. Frankly, I've never felt more attractive.' Sandra, 53, retailer.

'I don't feel old, but I'm lucky – I have my health and a fulfilling lifestyle. Too many women worry about losing their looks and that only makes things worse. When you're older, you can be just as attractive, but in a different way. Your character develops and it shows on your face. Life's a school and we're pupils in it. It's my zest for life that keeps me young.' Betty, 65, grandmother.

HOW THIS BOOK CAN HELP

There's no such thing as eternal youth – thank goodness. There's no cream or drug that can stop the clock, or instantly reverse the ageing process. But there are minor miracles that can help you look and feel so good about yourself that you'll radiate a natural, healthy, youthful zest for life.

Throughout the following chapters, we'll look out how to insure your health and beauty assets against the threat of premature ageing. Neither surgery nor costly salon treatments are included – these chapters deal with practical and realistic advice you can adapt to suit your lifestyle and turn into a lifetime's investment. As with all investment policies, the more you put into them in terms of care and dedication, the greater the rewards will be. It's never too late to start your anti-ageing programme, though the later you start the more work and time you'll have to put in to see results – and it's easy to feel discouraged unless there is some immediate improvement.

It's never too late to start your anti-ageing programme

That's why each chapter has its own 'Ten-minute tips' to give you a near-instant boost to get you looking and feeling younger faster. These are not so much corner cutters as fast-track back-ups to the main agenda, and you can choose the

> *You can choose the tips you need most to get you on track*

tips you need most to get you on track as and when you need them. Use as few or as many as you feel work for you each day. Make them into your own daily mini-programme; vary them throughout the week to fit in with the rest of your schedule; or tailor them to special occasions when you know you have to stay on the ball.

Because they're quick and easy, they'll encourage you to keep up the anti-ageing work. And because they give such fast results, you'll really notice the difference. Prepare yourself for compliments and enjoy!

ANTI-AGEING GAMEPLANS
LOOKING GREAT, WHATEVER YOUR AGE

THE THIRTIES

The first signs of ageing start to show. Your bone structure becomes more apparent as your skin 'slims' because production of supportive collagen and elastin proteins starts to slow. Crow's feet and smile and frown lines begin to show – especially if you sun-worshipped in your teens and twenties. You might also notice that your skin is slightly coarser and broken veins may have started to appear. Up to 90 per cent of sun damage is already done by the time you're 18, but the real effects don't show until now. The centre panel of your face may still be oily, though, and spots and adult acne may be triggered by stress, pregnancy and contraceptive and fertility drugs.

Skincare. Mild foaming cleansers suit both oily panels and dry surrounds. If your skin is very greasy, use an astringent or hydroxy acid-based tonic on the centre panel only. Use an oil-free moisturizer or, if your skin is slightly dry, a lightweight UV-screening moisturizer with antioxidant ingredients. If you've never used one before, invest in an eye cream. At night use your regular moisturizer or a lightweight antioxidant formula; or use a gentle hydroxy acid solution to prevent blackheads, regulate sebum flow and refine the skin surface. Use a gentle peeling mask a couple of times a week.

> *Invest in an eye cream*

Makeup. Oil-free foundation unifies skin and helps hide blemishes. Fresh neutral pink blush, dusted on cheek apples and browbones, warms and rounds the features. Light-reflective highlights on mid-lids and browbones 'open' eyes – choose shell pinks and gold-beige lights. Avoid block lid colour, but blend smudgy definition next to your lashes with a soft eyeshadow in chocolate or grey, plus brown-black lash-builder mascara. If the rest of your features stay soft and warm, you can opt for cool beige-pink lip tones.

Hair. First grey hairs may have already begun to show in your twenties. Demi-permanent tone-on-tone colour covers up to 50 per cent grey and lasts up to 20 washes. Use a mild, frequent-use shampoo that won't over-stimulate an oily scalp, but will refresh hair. A lightweight, oil-free conditioner polishes without weighing down bounce.

THE FORTIES

Genetic factors that programme how you age begin to kick in

for real. You may also begin to resemble a parent more strongly. Accumulated sun damage deepens frown, smile and crow's feet lines. Eye bags, loss of tone around the jawline, rings around the neck and a general loss of firmness all begin to show. Oil glands become enlarged and the T-zone pores start to dilate. Perversely, your skin may be dehydrated, but your oily centre panel may become even more apparent.

Skincare. Exfoliation is now crucial to your routine. AHA-based day and night treatments help keep pores free from debris, while refining surface coarseness. A vitamin A moisturizer may also help regulate sebum, stimulate collagen production and so preserve skin firmness. Serums applied directly to troublespots intensify the action of regular treatment creams and are especially useful after bouts of illness, stress or sun exposure. Use high-factor sunscreens regularly – there is evidence that skin can still go some way to repair itself if protected from further sun exposure. Choose firming eye gels and compresses to help ease lines and relieve shadows and morning puffiness. Face masks and 'instant' firmers are also brightening allies. Mild foams are still the best cleansers which dissolve makeup and grease without disrupting the skin's acid mantle. Use astringent toners on the centre panel only.

> *Exfoliation is now crucial to your routine*

Makeup. Avoid dull matt textures, but be wary of shimmer that highlights wrinkles. Opt for light-reflective foundations that unify the skintone and deflect dark shadows. Concentrate powder on the centre panel – never around the eyes, where it advertises lines. Blush is now a powerful ally – dust it over cheeks, browbones, on the brow near the hairline and along the jawline to soften your features and create a halo of warmth. Edit your eye makeup – what works best now is neutral, low-key shadow, simple definition along the lashlines and strictly no hard lines. Keep lashes 'clean' and groomed. For lips, avoid glosses that creep into lines around the lipline. Warm beige, rosewood and hot coral tones work hardest.

Hair. Now may be the time to consider a restyle. Shorter hair uplifts; face-framing highlights brighten the skintone and conceal increasingly grey hair. Short hair also looks fuller as it's easier to coax away from the scalp. Use a body-boosting styling aid to build volume and control and practise 'scrunching' hair dry to work life into your style. Cleanse with a mild, frequent use or moisturizing formula. A leave-in conditioner looks after tinted hair.

THE FIFTIES AND ONWARDS

There are now very tangible signs of ageing. Skin begins to thin and sag as collagen and elastin production slows dramatically. The first age spots may appear as melanin bundles clump and produce uneven pigmentation. Hormonal fluctuations throughout the menopause can trigger acne flare-up, but for the most part the skin rapidly loses its ability to retain moisture and so becomes dehydrated. This emphasizes lines and surface coarseness. Research suggests that HRT minimizes collagen breakdown after menopause and stimulates production of hyaluronic acid, the skin's own moisture-retaining connective tissue lubricant.

Skin. For daytime, moisturizing, firming vitamin A creams with sunscreens and antioxidant ingredients help protect against rapid deterioration. Overnight, vitamin A creams work overtime. Serums worn under regular moisturizers are face-saving intensives after sun, stress or illness. Skin resurfacing is still an issue but avoid AHA-based cleansers and moisturizers. Older skin is often thinner, more fragile, and prone to sensitivity.

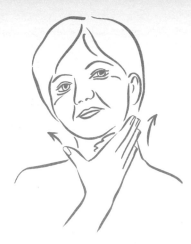

Gently buffing skin dry with a towel after cleansing exfoliates without irritation. If your skin feels tight after cleansing, change to a non-foaming 'wash' and gently massage off with damp cotton wool. When you need it, give your skin a soothing moisture boost with a mask. Pay extra attention to your neck, moisturizing liberally with a firming formula.

Makeup. Minimalism and subtlety are now your watchwords. A light-reflective treatment foundation and a warm tawny-pink or soft coral cream blush are your hardest-working items. A pale beige, demi-sheen eyeshadow opens up hooded eyes; the barest trace of brown powder shadow under lower lashes defines them. Replace fading lashcolour without overloading, using a brown mascara. If you need to 'flesh out' thinning lips, outline first with a neutral pencil, building slightly over the natural contour. Then fill in with a lipstick a hint warmer than your own lip tone.

Hair. Velcro rollers help to fill out fine hair by lifting it from the scalp;

> *Minimalism and subtlety are now your watchwords*

a medium-hold hairspray aimed at the roots holds the volume. Mousses boost body but some may prove 'scurfy' – choose conditioning formulas. Moisturize dry hair and scalp with a protein shampoo and conditioner. Revive freshness between washes with an anti-frizz serum which also polishes tinted and silver hair with a light-catching sheen.

YOUR TOP TEN PRIORITY AGE-BEATING TIPS

1 **Protect your skin.** Ninety per cent of wrinkles are caused by sun damage. A sunscreen is your first line of age defence.

2 **Keep to your ideal weight**. A plump face looks younger, but excess weight increases the risk of heart disease in later life by up to 25 per cent. If you're too thin, your face looks haggard and you increase your risk of osteoporosis. (See the chart, right, for your ideal weight.) Since your metabolism slows after 30 and is down by 4 per cent by 40, start reducing calories by 100 daily per decade.

3 **Keep moving.** Exercise reduces the risk of osteoporosis, heart disease and other age-related conditions. It controls weight and boosts immunity and mental alertness. T'ai Chi and yoga increase strength, flexibility, co-ordination and balance. Swimming lowers heart rate and detoxifies the body by boosting lymph circulation. Regular aerobic exercise boosts circulation and heart rate, bringing oxygen and colour to your skin.

4 **Give up smoking.** It robs the skin of oxygen, generates free radicals and is thought to hasten lines and wrinkles. It may also wreck your figure – studies suggest that smoke causes hormones to direct more fat to the stomach and middle regions. Worse, it increases the risk of breast, cervical and lung cancer.

5 **Rethink your hairdo.** Shorter hair 'uplifts' features and can

Is Your Weight Right For Your Height?

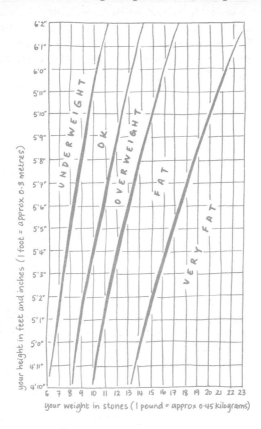

your height in feet and inches (1 foot = approx 0·3 metres)

your weight in stones (1 pound = approx 0·45 kilograms)

be as effective as a face lift. Softer, feathery styles are more flattering than geometrical cuts that take a lot to live up to. Make colour an ally. Rich vegetable rinses polish hair and conceal first grey; highlights near to your face lift and flatter your skintone.

6 Edit your makeup. Sticking to the same old look you had when you were 20 is the most ageing pitfall. Stay current –

and realistic. Ease up on eye makeup and major on warm lip and cheek tones that bring vitality to your face.

7 Dress well. Slightly fitted clothes give your figure structure and help conceal lumps and bumps better than baggy ones. Avoid relentless black or navy near your face – brighten it with a cream or pastel top. But too much beige looks bland – accessorize it with livelier but still natural tones like hot corals, salmon, ochre and rust. Avoid acid colours – limes and oranges and some yellows drain colour from your face.

8 Relax. Stress control dramatically reduces the risk of heart attack. Yoga, for example, relaxes your mind, encourages body awareness, and maintains suppleness, poise and muscle control. And sleep well – your body heals and regenerates overnight.

9 Welcome changes. Go with the flow. Remember, we never stop growing. Our potential is therefore huge!

10 Give yourself time – and go for it! It can take as little as ten minutes a day to start working on your act. Whatever your age, the results are incremental – they just get better and better.

CHAPTER 2

Skincare

Facing up to time

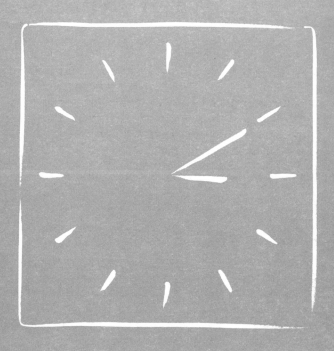

I t's no secret that your face is first to show your age. That's why efficient skincare is crucial to provide skin with the help it needs not to look older than it has to. As we get older, we can't get away with bad skin habits like we used to – neglect shows up fast in a dull complexion and hard, dry lines. But the right kind of care and protection gives skin the boost it needs to keep glowing on.

WHAT HAPPENS WHEN SKIN AGES?

Like the rest of our body tissue, skin gradually loses its youthful appearance and efficiency as part of the ageing process. The first signs of ageing begin to appear as early as our mid-thirties, but to limit the damage we should practise skin protection throughout life.

Changes in the dermis, the skin's lower layer, show up on the epidermis, or surface. Production of collagen and elastin, the foundation proteins, begins to slow, so the skin becomes thinner, losing its plumpness, firmness and elasticity. Think of collagen as the springs supporting a mattress. As these springs collapse and lose their symmetrical arrangement, the skin's foundation begins to crumble. On the surface, deeper lines, wrinkles and sagging start to appear.

Sluggish circulation means the complexion loses its glow and may seem paler and more drawn. Because the bloodstream nourishes cells less efficiently, they too become sluggish. In time, cell turnover can slow down by up to 50 per cent. Because new cells take longer to push up to the surface, dead flakes hang around longer, leaving the complexion dull and powdery-looking.

> *The first signs of ageing begin to appear as early as our mid-thirties*

This build-up of dead cells on the surface disturbs the skin's naturally protective barrier function, which helps to seal in vital moisture. Fluctuations in hormonal levels throughout our body lead to a reduced sebum output in skin, so the surface appears rougher, drier and less able to hold moisture. Chronic moisture loss leads to dehydration, and skin plumpness suffers even more. Dry skin may also become sensitive to irritation, and environmental extremes can worsen the damage.

ANTI-AGEING AGENTS

While it can't claim miracles or turn back the clock, efficient skincare can help you look younger for longer. Used regularly, a good anti-ageing cream can also ease the appearance of lines and wrinkles and give your complexion a more youthful, dewy finish. Despite skincare manufacturers' claims, whether or not cosmetic creams can substantially 'repair' wrinkles or 'lift' loose skin is still debatable. Only prescription drugs like Retin-A and Retinova (see below) have been clinically proven to radically smooth lines, but using the right cosmetic protection can help prevent them. The only problem is that there are so many formulas on the market that choosing is confusing. It can also be costly. So which are the anti-ageing ingredients that really pay their way? When you shop for anti-ageing creams, these ingredients should feature on your priority list:

MOISTURIZERS

More than anything, skin needs moisture – at least 60 per cent of its volume – to stay smooth, plump and translucent. Water keeps cells soft and permeable, so nutrients can enter and waste products are easily expelled. A moisturizer's basic job is to boost the skin's Natural Moisture Factor (NMF), help conserve fluid in the upper layers and prevent loss from deeper down. Sunlight, central heating, wind, cold and pollution all cause moisture loss, so moisturizers also strengthen the skin's barrier against environmental threat.

> *More than anything, skin needs moisture*

The stratum corneum – the skin's horny outer layer – is crucial to its barrier function. In young, healthy skin, natural oils and friendly flora preserve the slightly acid mantle that keeps keratin cells in the horny layer together. These overlapping dead skin cells form a scaly, water-resistant seal. But as skin ages, natural oil production slows and the skin surface becomes drier and less able to conserve moisture. Surface scales roughen and curl up, creating cracks in the barrier through which moisture escapes, while the defective surface barrier leaves deeper cells vulnerable to damage. As cell turnover also slows down, it takes longer for new cells to replace the dead ones. Moisturizers containing lipids such as ceramides help to strengthen the horny layer. Dermatologists agree that if this layer does its barrier job, the deeper layers where ageing begins stay protected and remain more able to fend for themselves.

SUNSCREENS

Sun is skin enemy Number 1. Whereas moderate doses allow the skin to synthesize vitamin D for healthy bones, dermatologists now estimate that 90 per cent of lines, wrinkles, sagging and coarsening are directly caused by ultraviolet light. Sun is also directly responsible for senile lentigenes – brown age spots which freckle the face, chest and hands and are among ageing's ugliest give-

Sunlight both ages skin and courts cancer

aways. Sunlight both ages skin and courts cancer. It used to be thought that only the 'burning' ultraviolet-B caused damage. Now it is known that whereas 95 per cent of these short-wave rays are absorbed by the epidermis, 80 per cent of so-called 'tanning' ultraviolet-A rays penetrate deep down to the dermis itself, attacking collagen and elastin as well as cell nuclei.

In the UK, 40,000 new cases of skin cancer are diagnosed each year. Left untreated, some can prove fatal. Dermatologists recommend a product with an SPF (Sun Protection Factor) no lower than 15 for health and serious anti-ageing protection. Make sure your cream has combined 'broad spectrum' UVA and UVB screens and wear it even in the city in dull weather. UVA light is constantly present year-round and can penetrate glass. If your moisturizer doesn't have a built-in SPF, apply a sun cream 20 minutes before you moisturize to allow the screen to sink into your skin.

ANTIOXIDANTS

Antioxidants are skincare's favourite troubleshooters because they work on ageing's most direct cause. Antioxidants mop up free radicals – super-oxygen molecules that latch onto weak cells. As members of the body's 'clean-up' squad free radicals aid natural tissue breakdown, but they can also get out of control – smoking, traffic fumes and sunlight all excite them. It's estimated that the DNA in every cell in the body comes under attack around 10,000 times daily from free radicals. They oxidize and harden lipids in the skin, meaning cells suffocate and starve because they can't absorb nutrients.

Antioxidants neutralize free radicals by giving them something to latch onto other than cells. They can then convert them to harmless compounds ready for natural elimination from the skin.

These days, it's hard to find an anti-ageing cream without one or all of the 'big three' antioxidants, vitamins A, C and E. Countless studies have shown how in the skin's upper layers the ACE team can have a protective equivalent of SPF 2 or 3, neutralizing free radical damage from sunlight and pollution. Vitamins A and C are also responsible for the synthesis of collagen and elastin – the 'plump and flex' proteins that keep skin springy and wrinkle-free. Some cosmetologists suggest the skin turns vitamin A into minute doses of retinoic acid – the active chemical of skin repair drugs Retin-A and Retinova (Renova). Vitamin E is also an excellent surface lubricant.

> *Vitamin E is an excellent surface lubricant*

Other useful antioxidants include zinc, copper, manganese, selenium and superoxide dismutase. Bioflavonoids in green tea extract combat inflammation. Recently, interest has been escalating around oligomeric proanthocyanadin complexes (OPCs), found mostly in grape-seed extracts. Said to be 50 times more effective than vitamin E and 20 times more potent than vitamin C, they are also known to protect against free radical damage to blood vessels and prevent the cross-linking of collagen, a major cause of loss of skin flexibility.

But the most exciting news to date is that an 18-month European study (part of the Supplemental Vitamin and Mineral Antioxidant Trial, or SU.VI.MAX) has now proved that daily application of creams containing antioxidants C and E both slows the formation of wrinkles by 23 per cent and can actually ease lines by 8 per cent. According to Daniel Maes, Vice President of Estée Lauder Research and Development Worldwide, who supplied the cream, regular antioxidant protection gives the skin a chance to reverse its own damage. That's one cosmetic claim to really listen to.

ALPHA AND BETA HYDROXY ACIDS

Also called fruit acids, AHAs exfoliate the skin by loosening the glue-like bonds that hold dead cells together on the surface. This boosts slow cell turnover and helps other skin-care ingredients to penetrate. AHAs are also said to help fade lines and pigment patches (age spots) and boost the skin's hyaluronic acid (moisture) quota. There is evidence they improve sun-tolerance up to an equivalent of SPF 2.5. Trials at the University of California in Los Angeles indicate they may even encourage collagen production.

High concentrations of highly acidic AHAs – especially the tiniest, highly penetrative glycolic acid molecule – can cause sensitive skin reactions. The newest cosmetic formulas use glycolic acid 'buffered' to an acid value nearer to that of the skin to miminize the risk. Other formulas use lactic acid, because its larger molecule has a strictly superficial action, so is less likely to provoke deeper irritation. Salicylic acid, a beta-hydroxy acid (BHA), is becoming increasingly popular, as it is far more easily tolerated even by sensitive skins. AHAs and BHAs work best on 35+ skin and results can be rewardingly rapid. They also unclog pores and help regulate oily, acne-prone skin.

SKIN DRUGS – ANTI-AGEING ON PRESCRIPTION

The only anti-ageing formulas clinically proven to reverse lines and wrinkles are prescription-only drugs based on a 'super' form of vitamin A. Brand-named Retin-A, retinoic acid was originally prescribed to treat acne, but patients also noticed their skin had fewer lines, age spots and pigmentation patches and looked generally firmer, plumper and brighter. On the surface, retinoic acid works by exfoliating dead cells and revealing a clearer texture. Deeper down in the dermis, it plumps up the skin by triggering new formation of collagen and elastin and strengthens weakened blood vessels.

The drawbacks are that higher concentrations of retinoic acid give the best results, but pose the worst risk of swelling, soreness, peeling and redness. In addition, skin becomes far more UV-sensitive, and has to be protected with a sunblock worn over Retin-A at all times. Retinoids have also been linked with the risk of birth defects, should creams be used in early pregnancy, although recent tests have failed to substantiate this. Retin-A is available as a gel, lotion or cream in several strengths. The strongest and most likely to cause irritancy is 0.1 per cent; the mildest is 0.025 per cent.

Many dermatologists like to start patients off on low concentrations and gradually work upwards as the skin builds tolerance. After around a year of regular use, the dose and frequency can be reduced to a maintenance level. However, if you stop using the product the lines simply come back.

A milder version, Retinova (Renova in the US), is now also available from dermatologists and cosmetic surgery clinics. Containing 0.05 per cent tretinoin (a form of retinoic acid), its very mild formula is aimed specifically at reversing sun damage, with a lower irritancy risk. For women who don't want to face surgery or laser treatment, this could well be the key to regaining smoother, firmer skin.

WHEN ENOUGH IS ENOUGH!

Can you have too much of a good thing? Smothering the skin with TLC can hinder its ability to look after itself. Don't overdo it. Moderation is better for your skin and your purse!

MOISTURE MANAGEMENT

Don't overload, says New York celebrity dermatologist Patricia Wexler. Older women with dry skin tend to slap on heavy creams, but too much, she says, sags the skin and can cause blocked pores. During the day, ease up on the layers – if your foundation has an in-built moisturizer, you may not need such a rich formula underneath.

Moderation is better for your skin and your purse!

CAREFUL CLEANSING

Dermatologists warn that obsessional cleansing – say, three or four times a day – especially with an alkaline product, can seriously affect the skin's acid mantle. The result is chronic dryness and iritation, which as well as hastening lines may also lead to conditions like eczema. Be careful with AHA-based cleansers, too. Some dermatologists worry that since cleansing already loosens dead surface cells, AHAs may also loosen deeper cells, leaving the skin open to sensitivity and product overload. If you're worried, restrict AHA cleansers to two or three times a week or avoid them altogether.

DO YOU REALLY NEED A NIGHT CREAM?

There's no reason why you shouldn't use your daytime moisturizer overnight. Obviously, your skin doesn't need a sunscreen now but, say experts, night creams may deliver extra benefits. During sleep, the body secretes 70 per cent of its daily dose of human growth hormone, the chemical impetus skin needs to run repairs and maintain cell health and vitality. A boost in metabolic activity between 1 a.m. and 3 a.m. also means the skin's energy chemicals peak and cell division increases. Sophisticated night creams claim that as

| **Night creams may deliver extra benefits** | well as offering overnight protection against moisture loss, they can work with the skin's repair rhythms, supplementing the energy cells need to create a smooth, firm complexion. |

How do they do it? Night-time formulas are more emollient than daycreams and designed to soften skin for longer periods. Since research shows that skin is more permeable overnight, active ingredients can penetrate more easily. 'If you apply night cream when you go to bed, treatment molecules have time to penetrate to where and when the cells can really use them,' says Estée Lauder's Daniel Maes. Since vitamins A, C and E may take a minimum of six hours to penetrate, using an antioxidant cream overnight is the best way of ensuring your skin stays protected next day, he adds.

TROUBLESHOOTING SKIN PROBLEMS

No matter what type of skin they have, few women are satisfied with what they've got – and as age takes its toll the flaws only seem to get bigger. Nevertheless, there's a lot you can do to alleviate skin problems of all types.

OILY SKIN

In theory, sebum output lessens with age. Hormones control the sebaceous (oil) glands and testosterone (the 'male' hormone), which surges in both sexes at puberty, can also influence skin in mid-life. According to Dr Anthony Chu, consultant dermatologist to the UK Acne Support Group, stress-linked testosterone is a common cause of acne in career women. Oestrogen counteracts testosterone, so some contraceptive pills control oily skin and acne. But the progestogen-only 'mini-pill' can cause acne as the body metabolizes progestogen into testosterone. On a practical level, New York dermatologist Patricia Wexler believes oily skin should neither be punished nor pampered. Alcohol-based astringents dissolve oil but they also can

Stress-linked testosterone is a common cause of acne in career women

strip out moisture, causing extra production of oil if the skin thinks it is lacking. Many oily skin ranges now use alternative oil-blotters in toners, so minimizing the risk of aggravation. AHA-based cosmetics can help regulate moderately oily skin. Salicylic acid (BHA) is an effective exfoliant degreaser in toners and spot control lotions. For more stubborn spots, use a benzoyl peroxide treatment, keeping it well away from surrounding skin. To keep skin comfortable, use an oil-free moisturizer on drier zones only.

DRY SKIN

When oil production drops after the menopause, skin loses its ability to retain moisture. A tendency to dryness is inherited; central heating, air conditioning and temperature swings don't help. Ultraviolet light also disrupts cellular cohesion, unpicking the tight defensive mesh of cells in the epidermis, so moisture escapes through loopholes.

Dermatologists urge that it is vital to keep dry skin adequately moisturized to prevent irritation and infection. An excessively dry skin could be an early warning of atopic eczema, says Dr Ian White, consultant dermatologist at St

Creams don't have to be greasy to work

Thomas's Hospital, London. Gentle exfoliation helps keep the surface smooth and moisture-receptive. Creams don't have to be greasy to work – choose the texture that feels most comfortable and reapply it whenever your skin feels tight. Humidifiers in homes and offices help keep the air moist and prevent dry, itchy skin.

SENSITIVE SKIN

As many as 60 per cent of British women claim to have sensitive skin. Pale, fair, dry skin is most likely to be sensitive. But what's the difference between sensitive and allergic? Sensitivity can be caused by sun, wind, rough handling, even water. Redness, itching, swelling and stinging are rapid responses – but the same triggers may not provoke repeat reactions. An allergic reaction, however, happens each time the skin comes in contact with the trigger. Perfumes, preservatives, colourings, detergents and surfactants and some sunscreens are all common cosmetic allergens. Responses vary, but blisters, cracking, oozing, scaling and redness are all typical. Even if you react to one known allergen you won't necessarily flare up at them all, but you will react each time you contact your trigger. It's thought that sensitivity can lead to full-blown allergy. Years of chronic irritation weakens the skin and causes significant ageing. Hypo-allergenic and sensitive skincare ranges exclude high-risk allergens and irritants, while containing calming and strengthening agents. Even so, do a patch test before you buy a new product. Apply a penny-sized dab on your inside upper arm and cover for 24 hours. Then repeat. If redness or irritation occurs, stop using the product.

> *Do a patch test before you buy a new product*

AGE SPOTS

Senile lentigenes are caused by a lifetime's exposure to UV rays. As we age, melanin pigment becomes less evenly distributed and forms in clumps, like giant freckles. They're most obvious on areas which are constantly exposed – especially hands, arms and chest as well as the face. Preparations containing 2 per cent hydroquinone (the permitted EC 'safe' level) fade age

Liquorice extract helps prevent age spots forming

spots by dissolving melanin granules just beneath the skin's surface. Liquorice extract helps prevent age spots forming by inhibiting tyrosinase, the enzyme responsible for melanin synthesis. But above all, always wear a hand cream with a high sun protection factor.

FACIAL HAIR

Falling oestrogen levels around the menopause mean androgens responsible for body hair growth may become more active. Hereditory factors and stress may also play a role. Shadowy moustaches and chin whiskers are embarrassing – they look 'murky' and feel rough. Bleaching them isn't ideal, as the hairs tend to coarsen and stick out against darker skin tones. Plucking is an easy way of coping with just a few regulars – there's no evidence hair grows back stronger – or use a gentle facial depilatory. Creams that inhibit regrowth contain agents that 'starve' hairs by blocking delivery of nutrients to the roots. For a long-term solution, electrolysis can block regrowth by destroying hair roots but it is painful. Lasers have proved effective, but can't be used on fair hair or dark skin. A new treatment using Intense Pulsed Light heats individual hairs, so roots are destroyed. Suitable for all hair and skin colours, it's no more painful than pins and needles and can reduce hair growth by 50 per cent in a single treatment. After that, regrowth is rare.

EYES – WHY THEY'RE A DELICATE ZONE

The eye surrounds are the first areas to register signs of age. They develop lines faster than the rest of the face because continual movement – blinking, smiling and frowning – stresses the thin, delicate skin. There are also fewer oil glands around the eyes, making the skin there a traditionally dry zone. Yet the lightest moisturizers are the most effective carers.

FROWN LINES AND CROW'S FEET

> *Use a light-textured eye cream with a built-in sun filter*

Expression lines are inevitable – try really smiling without wrinkling your eyes! However, screwing up the eyes against bright light worsens UV-damage and hastens crow's feet. Use a light-textured eye cream with a built-in sun filter. Always wear sunglasses in bright light – they help prevent eye damage, such as cataracts, too.

PUFFINESS AND UNDER-EYE BAGS

These result from decreased muscle tone in the lower lid and a herniation of the underlying fatty layer. Puffiness, or oedema, is due to poor lymphatic circulation. Excess fluid floods the spaces between fatty tissue, particularly after long periods lying down – hence early-morning puffy eyes.

Choose a firming eye-care formula with a temporary tightening agent such as squalene or shark cartilage. Avoid rich, oily textures, which overload thin skin and puff it up even more. Gels have a natural tightening effect and won't stray into the eye itself – crucial for contact lens wearers. Apart from exercise, which kick-starts lymph drainage, the most effective way of minimizing puffiness is to sleep with your pillow raised.

DARK CIRCLES

These occur when stress, fatigue, chronic UV exposure and persistent swelling weaken delicate blood capillaries to breaking point. Exhaustion and illness hamper circulation in the surrounding facial skin, so a washed-out complexion also highlights dark circles under eyes. Exercise oxygenates surrounding skin, so the 'glow' makes shadows less noticeable. In creams, the latest deshadowing active ingredient is vitamin K, which strengthens microcapillaries, preventing rupture and leakage of blood and lymph – a key cause of puffy, bruised-looking skin.

GENTLE-TOUCH EYE CARE

Cleansing.   Never rub or stress delicate skin around the eyes. Always use a special eye cleanser formulated to dissolve eye makeup easily, especially hard-to-shift long-lasting and waterproof formulas. If you wear contact lenses avoid very oily formulas, which are difficult to rinse. Soak cleanser into cotton-wool pads and rest on closed lids for a few seconds, then gently wipe downwards and outwards. Repeat until the pads are clear.

> *Never rub or stress delicate skin around the eyes*

Protecting.   Keep regular moisturizers away from the eye area – most are too heavy. Choose light, semi-fluid creams or gels that sink in fast and don't creep into the eyes. To prevent overloading the lids, pat gently around the eye orbits. Experts say that most formulas eventually reach the lids too, so the whole area is treated.

TEN-MINUTE TIP

Wake up sore, tired eyes

Tone and refresh sore, puffy eyes after too much sun, sleep or VDU work. Keep an eye mask or used camomile tea bags in the fridge. Rest on closed lids.

Soothe dry, strained, gritty eyes and clear redness. Carefully hydrate eyes with vitaminized moisturizing drops. Avoid astringent formulas and choose drops that are pH balanced to tears. To minimize stinging and flooding, gently pull down the lower lid with a fingertip, look up and squeeze the drops in. Rest with closed lids. Wash your hands first and don't allow the nozzle to touch your eyes. Always throw away drops after the 'use-by' period (usually within one month) to avoid the risk of bacterial infection.

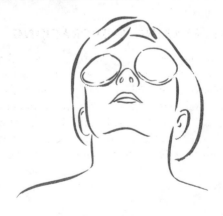

LIPS – PRESERVING THE POUT

Lips have few sebaceous glands, are sensitive to low humidity and lack pigment to defend themselves from sun damage. Consequently, they chap and flake easily. Even more of a problem is wrinkling around the lip contours – a tell-tale sign of ageing. Here's how to prevent the worst.

WRINKLES AND PUCKERING

Just as our skin loses plumpness with age, so do our lips. Gums too shrink gradually, providing less padding to prevent puckering. Like eyes, lips are highly mobile. But smoking is probably the worst cause of wrinkles, since the mechanical action, plus free radical activity, significantly weakens the contour. Firming 'lip lift' products contain moisturizers, plus polymers that seal the lip surrounds, temporarily plumping and tightening the lips. Since most contain regular anti-ageing benefits, you can wear them round the clock as well as under lipstick to prevent feathering.

DRYNESS, FLAKING AND CRACKING

Use a conditioning salve on its own or under lipstick to protect lips from moisture loss. Those with sunscreens are preferable, since herpes simplex (cold sore) blisters are triggered by heat and sunlight. Salves and sticks containing tea tree oil help to prevent this, while speeding the healing of cracks and chaps. Overnight, slather on Vaseline – it really is the best softening, moisture-sealing agent for dry, rough lips.

TEN-MINUTE TIP

Dry lip rescue

To plump lips and get rid of flakes, smother the entire mouth area with Vaseline and leave for five minutes. With a soft, damp toothbrush, gently scrub away loosened flakes. The circulation boost temporarily firms lips and leaves them rosy. Rinse, pat dry and slick on salve.

CLEANSING – IS IT SAFE TO WASH YOUR FACE?

Really, it's down to comfort, convenience and how clean your skin feels. If you're like Liz Taylor and Claudia Schiffer, you won't allow water near your skin. If you're like me, life's too short to mess around with lotions. So unless your skin's so sensitive that water stings, washing has a lot going for it.

Avoid basic soap, though – it's far too alkaline and acts like a solvent to your skin's natural oil. Choose an acid (pH) balanced bar or foaming cleanser that respects your skin's natural acidity (around pH 5.5–5.6) and is less likely to leave your skin feeling tight and degreased. Foaming cleansers are easier to rinse off than creams and lotions – a considerable advantage, since stale makeup traces and alkaline chemicals like emulsifiers and surfactants left on the skin can cause dryness and irritation. But do rinse well – use several splashings of running water.

Avoid basic soap

Lukewarm is the ideal temperature for dissolving suds without damaging fragile skin capillaries. A final cold water splash gives the skin a temporary firming glow by sending the circulation rushing to the skin surface.

Still love your lotion? You can rinse off your cream and lotion with warm water, too. Alternatively, use a damp flannel/washcloth to gently but firmly wipe around angles and corners until they test absolutely clear.

How often do you need to cleanse? Over-zealous cleansing disrupts the skin's acid mantle, making it more irritant-prone. But if you wear makeup, cleansing before bed is vital. Leaving occlusive grime on skin overnight can inhibit the penetration of useful ingredients in overnight moisturizers. It's also seriously bad skin hygiene, says Daniel Maes, Vice-President of Research and Development for Estée Lauder Worldwide: 'Long-term poor cleansing habits create blackheads, acne lesions and bumps under the skin.' In the morning, a lighter cleanse removes stale cream, sebum and perspiration and prepares the skin for fresh moisture and makeup. Besides, would your face look awake without it?

TONING – DO YOU NEED TO?

Not really, say dermatologists, who worry that women use toners as cleansing back-ups to remove whatever's left. Their opinion is that if your cleanser is efficient you shouldn't need a toner. But manufacturers argue that slightly acidic toners help the skin to quickly normalize its natural pH, which cleansing may have disturbed. Fair enough, toners do soothe and refresh the skin, and some contain light moisturizing as well as calming agents. So treat them as comforters, but never cleansers.

EXFOLIATION – THE ANTI-AGEING BASIC

Always gently rub up and out against the direction of your wrinkles

Polishing off dead surface cells is skincare's most basic anti-ageing essential. Exfoliation smoothes wrinkles, softens the skin surface, boosts circulation and clears pores of accumulated debris. But how do you do it well?

Dermatologists warn that over-zealous buffing with abrasive pads and scratchy granules can irritate and damage skin. Choose a product with smoothly rounded polymer microbeads that lift dead skin without scratching. Or use a latex-based 'gommage' which dries on the skin so that you can gently rub it off with your fingertips.

Always gently rub up and out against the direction of your wrinkles. Avoid the eye zone and steer clear of areas with broken veins and blemishes. How often should you exfoliate? Every other day if your skin is tolerant; otherwise, two or three times weekly.

Passive exfoliation with AHA products prevents dead skin build-up. A gentle buff with a face brush or towel after washing finally removes flakes that AHAs have already loosened. Some beauty experts still recommend you exfoliate manually a couple of times a week, but dermatologists warn that since AHAs can sensitize, manual scrubbing on top can cause serious irritation. If your skin is already sensitive, choose an anti-irritant formula and don't mix your methods.

INSTANT FIRMERS AND BRIGHTNESS BOOSTERS

Do you believe in miracles? These anti-ageing agents promise instant results, but not all of their benefits last.

LIFTERS

These are usually fairly fine fluids with firming agents such as polymers that smooth, firm and cling to the skin surface. The clinging effect can be very slightly irritating, so bringing the blood rushing to the surface – hence the glow. The effect is temporary, but gives a satisfyingly smooth base for makeup and an emergency boost for dull skin.

SMOOTHERS

Serums are recommended by beauty therapists after excess summer sun, illness and winter's extreme conditions. They are concentrates of the active ingredients in the cosmetic ranges they belong to. Worn under regular moisturizer, they are meant to give the skin an extra 'fix'. Their ultra-light texture means they sink in fast, giving the skin a fresher, more dewy look. Unless your skin is very dry, the newest generation of moisturizing, lifting serums may be all you need, especially under makeup.

MASKS

These increase the skin circulation – hence the afterglow. Clay-based masks draw sebum and debris from the skin surface, help keep pores unplugged, are mildly exfoliative and can have a slight tightening effect.

Moisturizing masks are deeply soothing and can be a real relief to sore, taut skins, leaving the surface better hydrated and more supple. The effects are usually only temporary, but the feelgood factor may see you through an evening. You can turn your moisturizer into an emergency mask by applying it extra-thick, leaving it for 10 minutes, then tissuing off the excess.

TEN-MINUTE TIP

The fast-track facial

Give your skin a pick-me-up before a big event.

Cleanse. Whisk the skin with a soft brush and cleanser to detox pores, exfoliate and boost circulation. Rinse and blot the skin damp, not dry. Two minutes.

Massage. Do one complete facial circuit (see massage movements, page 46). Use a nourishing oil or cream. Three minutes.

Mask. Apply directly over your moisturized skin to encourage it to penetrate further. Soak cotton pads or cold compresses in eye makeup remover. Relax, lids closed, for four minutes. Remove mask, rinse and tone. Thirty seconds.

Moisturize. Use your regular day or night formula. Thirty seconds.

CHAPTER 3

Facial exercise
Lifting, not letting go

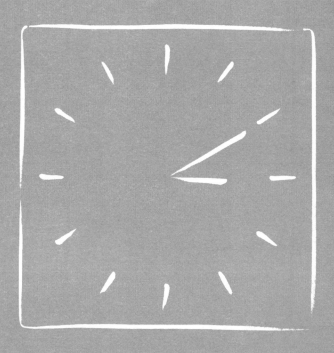

Do facial exercises work? The theory behind them seems plausible enough. If the muscles underlying our facial structure stay toned and tight, the skin will look firmer too. Pulling faces in a mirror seems an extreme and eccentric way of maintaining face, yet 'grimacing gurus' say these exercise systems go further than face lifts to maintain youthful facial firmness, because they help to prevent the problems that underly skin ageing.

Of the face's 57 muscles, we probably use only a few regularly. With age, the muscles flatten and elongate from lack of use and succumb to gravity. Just as skin loses its elasticity, bone, muscle and subcutaneous fat under our skin diminish. In effect, our faces get that bit smaller. The obvious result is loose, sagging skin that no longer seems to fit.

Carole Maggio, who devised the Facercise system of facial exercises, argues that cosmetic surgery is a fairly superficial way of dealing with these symptoms of ageing. In her view, surgical lifts are expensive, short-lived and can leave the face looking unnaturally taut. Exercise, however, tackles causes like weak underlying muscle and poor-quality microcirculation and is an inexpensive way of maintaining firm, glowing and naturally youthful skin. Within three weeks of beginning a programme you'll notice a difference around your facial contours, and because your circulation is improving, your complexion will look fresher and rosier, maintains Maggio.

Some dermatologists seem to agree with her. Dr Wilma Bergfield, President of the American Academy of Dermatology, concedes that reasonable facial exercise may improve and certainly can't damage the skin's appearance, while Beverly Hills surgeon Dr Lawrence Birnbaum believes exercising not only benefits patients' skin before and after surgery, it may actually go some way towards lifting poor tone without resorting to an operation. In the UK, Dr David Fenton of St John's Institute of Dermatology at St Thomas's Hospital feels facial exercises may have benefited some of his patients. He believes they are a cheaper, more practical and possibly more effective alternative to so-called non-surgical face-lift techniques which use electrical stimuli to 'twitch' muscles taut.

Fancy giving them a shot? Start your workout relaxed, with a clean face, in a warm, very private room away from prying eyes. You'll find the facial flexes exercises easier if your skin is comfortably moisturized. You can do the system any time, but first thing in the morning is best, to help chase away puffiness and 'wake up' your skin tone. At the very least, you'll start the day with a smile.

TOP TEN FACE-FIRMERS

Repeat each sequence three times

STREAMLINE A DOUBLE CHIN

1 With a closed, relaxed mouth, jut your chin forwards and slightly upwards.
2 Rest your elbow on a table and balance your chin on your clenched fist. Slide your lower lip up and over your top lip.
3 Press the tip of your tongue against the roof of your mouth, behind your top teeth. Increase the pressure over a count of five. Hold.

4 Slowly release the pressure over a count of five.

FIRM A SAGGING JAWLINE AND NECKLINE

1 Jut your chin upwards so that the front of your neck is taut.
2 Push your lower lip over your top lip towards your nose.
3 Keep your neck stretched. Slowly smile, pulling your mouth corners upwards and outwards over a count of five.
4 Hold for another five and stroke the jawline upwards with the flats of your hands.
5 Return slowly to the start over a count of five, gradually releasing your lip hold.

SMOOTH FOREHEAD LINES

1 Rest your elbows on the table and place your fingertips along your hairline.
2 Gently push your brow upwards and hold it against the bone.
3 Keep your head erect and look straight ahead. Bring your brow down in five movements using your forehead muscles, working against the resistance of your fingers, gradually closing your eyes.
4 Hold the downward pull for a count of three, then slowly release. Repeat three times.

LIFT A HEAVY BROW

1 Place your index fingers along your mid-forehead, parallel to your eyebrows, fingertips facing.
2 Press your fingers down to around 1cm ($^1/_2$ inch) above your brows.
3 Push your eyebrows up towards your fingers, then relax. Repeat ten times.
4 Raise your eyebrows again and press your fingers down.

Hold and do mini push-ups with your eyebrows until you feel a tight pressure building up.

5 Hold your eyebrows upwards and count to 20. Release.

TONE DROOPY EYELIDS

1 Look straight ahead. Curve your index fingers under your eyebrows.

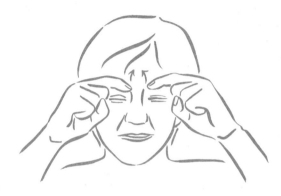

2 Push up your eyebrows and hold them firmly against the bone.
3 Close your lids very slowly, feeling the pull down from brow to lashes.
4 Squeeze your eyelids together tightly. Hold for a count of five.
5 Release the squeeze over a count of five.
6 Open your eyes and relax.

PREVENT PUFFY UNDER-EYE BAGS

1 Looking ahead, raise your eyebrows, then slowly raise your lower lids in five movements.
2 Close your eyes gently and squeeze the lids together. Hold

for a count of five, then slowly relax.

3 With your eyes still closed, slowly relax the lower lid muscles in five movements.

4 Open your eyes and relax.

STRENGTHEN THE LIP MUSCLES

1 Open your mouth slightly – about 2.5cm (1 inch).

2 Lower your jaw in eight slow movements. At the same time, gradually move your mouth corners inwards. Your mouth should then form an oval, your jaw should be dropped and your lips should feel taut.

3 Hold for a count of five, then relax your top lip in eight slow movements.

SMOOTH UPPER LIP WRINKLES

1 Rest your elbows on a table and look ahead. Place your thumbs under your top lip, the thumbnails resting against your gums. Your thumbs should point towards your eye pupils.

2 Gently move your upper lip muscles towards your thumbs in eight small movements.

3 With your upper lip pressed against your thumbs, hold for a count of five.

4 Keep your thumbs still and release your muscles in eight slow movements.

STRENGTHEN THE LOWER LIP AND CHIN MUSCLES

1 Keep your teeth about 2.5cm (1 inch) apart. Hook the first joint of your index fingers behind your lower lip, with your fingernails slightly away from your lower teeth and gums.

2 Move your lower lip muscles against the resistance of your

fingers, in eight movements.

3 With your muscles firmly pressed against your fingers, hold for a count of five.

4 Keep your fingers still and release your muscles in eight movements.

SMOOTH NOSE-TO-MOUTH LINES

1 Open your mouth into a long oval by pulling your upper and lower lips away from each other.

2 Use your upper lip only to pull your mouth corners up into a smile and at the same time wrinkle your nose.

3 Push your upper lip down hard against your teeth until you feel the pull at the sides of your nose.

4 Hold until it tingles, then slowly release.

Exercising for success

Sick of being told to cheer up? Loss of skintone and deep creaselines can give your face a sad, heavy look. Over time, facial exercises can help you reinvent your expression without moving a muscle! These are some of the things they can help you do.

- Give your skintone a glow
- Open up your eyes
- Get rid of puffiness
- Make lips look plumper, firmer, sexier
- Smooth lines and creases
- Firm up jowls and strengthen your jawline
- Tone your chin and neckline
- Allow your face to look relaxed – not grumpy or miserable.

TEN-MINUTE TIP: WAKE UP YOUR FACE!

This energizing exercise helps to dissolve signs of strain and tiredness by boosting the circulation to facial tissue. Do it any time your skin needs an extra glow.

- Lie down and pull the upper and lower lips apart into a long oval.
- Press your upper lip firmly down against your teeth.
- Use the corners of your mouth to smile, then relax. Repeat ten times.
- On smile ten, use extra energy to pull upper and lower lips even further away from each other. Hold for a count of 30, then relax.
- Now repeat, raising your head 2.5cm (1 inch) from the pillow. Hold for a count of 30.
- Repeat the entire sequence three times.

CHAPTER 4

Facial massage
Smoothing the years away

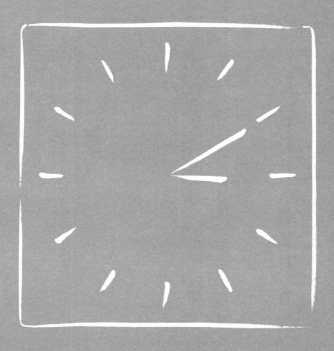

Massage improves the circulation and lymph drainage, leaving your skin looking fresher, less puffy and more glowing. Regular gentle stroking helps sweep away tension frowns and furrows by relieving stressed facial muscles and easing headaches and tiredness.

Massage is also an integral part of a facial. Therapists believe that a warm, relaxed skin is more receptive to treatment. During deep cleansing, for example, 'looser' pores are more likely to expel sebum plugs and debris. Cream 'sinks in' more easily, too, so massage helps the deeper penetration of nourishing, balancing agents. In salon facials, massage usually prepares the skin for the face mask, or 'intensive' stage, but you don't have to go the full facial monty to enjoy the benefit of

> *Massage is an integral part of a facial*

massage. Use the technique to improve the efficiency of your face creams, especially last thing at night when you need to relax most and can really go to town on deep moisturizing.

TEN-STEP TONIC MASSAGE

Massage your face three or four times a week, or whenever you find time. Always work on a clean, warm, moisturized skin. You can also incorporate these massage movements into a weekly home facial.

1 Use the backs of your hands alternately to stroke upwards from collarbone to chin. Tilt your head to the left and stroke the right side of your neck then repeat on the other side. Stroke firmly to stimulate the circulation and keep your neck young-looking.

2 Pinch along your jawline, using your thumbs and the knuckles of your index fingers. Start under your chin and work out towards your ears. Pinch close to the bone so you don't stretch the skin. This may help to prevent a double chin.

3 Slap gently under your chin with the backs of your hands, at the same time keeping your tongue curled back in your mouth to exercise the throat muscles.

4 Make an 'O' shape with your mouth and curl your lips tightly over your teeth. With your index fingers, make small circular pressures over your chin and round your mouth. Continue the pressures while you make exaggerated vowel shapes – ah, ee, ay, oh, oo – with your mouth. This helps prevent wrinkles around the lip contours.

5 Stroke from the corners of your mouth to your ears, using one hand per cheek.

6 With one hand following the other, stroke up your forehead from the bridge of your nose to your hairline. Keep your eyes closed and relaxed.

7 Massage the muscles between your eyebrows to ease frown lines. Place both index fingertips on the bridge of your nose and make short, firm strokes upwards, across, then diagonally.

8 With your fingertips, make circular pressures all over your forehead. Work from the bridge of your nose to your temples, covering your whole forehead right up to your hairline. Then soothe your forehead with gentle strokes from the centre to the temples. Finish by lightly pressing the temples.

9 Circle round your eyes with your middle fingertips. Stroke firmly from the bridge of your nose outwards over your

eyebrows. Press on the temples, then stroke very lightly under your eyes, sweeping outwards to the temples.
10 Pinch along your eyebrows from the centres to the temples. Gently press into the indentations in the browbones, just under the eyebrows where the bridge of the nose begins.

The right touch

Different massage movements have specific anti-ageing benefits. Vary your touch to give your face the full treatment, or customize your massage into a deeply relaxing or invigorating experience. Use brisk movements for a morning wake-up, say, or slow, soothing strokes for an evening calm-down. Remember – never drag or force your skin. Even firm pressure should also be gentle – never sharp, prodding or painful.

- Stroking improves circulation, relaxes tense muscles and soothes nerves. Slow movements calm, brisk movements stimulate.
- Kneading and pinching with fingers and thumbs gently stretches and relaxes tense muscles. This movement also improves circulation and therefore the absorption of nutrients via the bloodstream as well as the elimination of waste matter. Light kneading affects the skin and top layer of muscles; deep kneading affects deeper muscles.
- Tapping is usually done on the face with the pads of the fingertips, in a light 'drumming' action. This helps to stimulate lymph drainage and usually happens towards the end of a massage as it has an invigorating, stimulating and 'wake-up' effect.
- Pressure is also used to stimulate acupressure, or energy points on the face. Deep, gentle pressure with the fingertips eases muscular tension and activates circulation and lymph drainage.

FRIENDLY PRESSURE THAT MELTS TENSION

Pressure points are central to Shiatsu, or acupressure, a Japanese massage system that stimulates them to remove energy blocks and so improve vitality freeflow. These pressure, or energy, points occur where muscle, tissue and bone meet. They're fairly easy to find – press them and they produce a 'sweet pain' sensation, quite different to that of the surrounding skin. Massage the pressure points below to soothe pain and rid your face of stress signs. Use the fleshy pads of your second or third fingertips to gently press and vibrate for a count of ten, then release and repeat until tension eases.

Location 1: four points running in a line from the mid-hairline just above your forehead to the crown of your head.
Relieves: headaches and hangovers.

Location 2: a small dent at the centre of each eyebrow.
Relieves: headaches and migraines.

Location 3: between the eyebrows.
Relieves: headaches and migraine.

Location 4: on the rim of each cheekbone, directly below the eye pupil when you are looking straight ahead.
Relieves: headaches and migraines.

Location 5: just below the end of each eyebrow, level with the outer corner of the eyes.
Relieves: headaches and migraines.

Location 6: in the inner corner of each eye.
Relieves: sinus pain and eyestrain.

Location 7: in the grooves either side of the nose, where the upper lip ends and the nostrils begin.
Relieves: nasal congestion, sinus pain, toothache and facial tension.

Location 8: in the centre of the lip-to-nose grooves, above the cupid's bow.
Relieves: hunger pangs – useful if you're dieting.

Getting well oiled

Light oils can give better slip and minimize drag more efficiently than basic moisturizers, which often tend to sink in. Use a neat oil that suits your skin type, or add aromatherapy oils to turn your massage into a skin-balancing treatment.

Greasy or blemished skin. 3 drops each of lemon and bay in 30 drops of soya or grapeseed oil.

Dry, devitalized and mature skin. 3 drops each of patchouli, sandalwood and ylang ylang in 30 drops of wheatgerm oil.

Sensitive or puffy skin. 2 drops each of lavender and sandalwood in 20 drops of sesame or jojoba oil.

Puffy eye rescue

If you wake up puffy, here's how to help boost lymphatic drainage and disperse the trapped fluids that cause the 'hamster eye' look.

- Using your fingertips, lightly circle the eye orbits, following the contour of the sockets.
- Then, more firmly (but still gently), stroke several times from the bridge of the nose out across the eyebrows.
- Finally, use the first three fingertips of both hands to tap very lightly along the cheekbone ridge. Use a light 'drumming' action as if you're playing a piano and work from the inner to the outer eye corners.

TEN-MINUTE TIP

Calming palming

Not so much a massage, more a helping hand or two. Called palming, this very basic but wonderfully soothing technique refreshes tired eyes after VDU use, clears the mind, eases headaches and relaxes taut, tense facial muscles. Use it any time – several times a day, if you feel the need. You can also use palming to calm your face ready for massage. Afterwards, you'll look much more relaxed and less lined and drawn.

- Sit comfortably at a table or desk.
- Rest your palms over your face, fingers on forehead and heels of hands on chin.
- Hold for a moment, press gently, then slowly draw your hands out towards your ears, as if you're smoothing away tension.
- Repeat these gentle pressures at intervals of a few minutes until your ten minutes is up.

CHAPTER 5

A fresh approach
to makeup

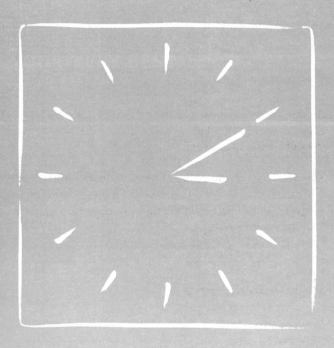

Using makeup is cheating – and it works! On a bad day, its feelgood factor boosts us out of the blues by emphasizing our good points and hiding the ones we'd rather not see. A touch of colour helps us enjoy the way we look and a little goes a very long way. It's the next best thing to a youth drug – and it's all good creative fun.

HOW TO GET OUT OF A MAKEUP RUT

Do you feel your face isn't working, but can't see why? According to makeup artist Bobbi Brown, these are warning signs of a major makeup rut:

- If you try to re-create favourite looks from past photographs.
- If you're devastated when your favourite lipstick or shadow is discontinued, or try to stockpile.
- If you feel naked without mascara and eyeliner.
- If you always line your lips with dark brown pencil.
- If you wear the same lipstick everywhere.
- If you labour over your look.
- If you always, always wear makeup.
- And, most importantly, if you haven't changed it in the last five years.

Anything here seem familiar? Your face is changing and so should your makeup strategy. Here's how to reassess.

Junk the dross. Anything you haven't used in the past year obviously isn't working for you, but don't experiment or panic – buy new makeup when you're feeling dreary. That's when a reassuring, tried and trusted look will give you confidence the most.

Adjust your look. Rethink your makeup if you have a new hair cut or colour. Going lighter, say, means your makeup colours should go fresher, not heavier.

Study form. Check fashion and beauty magazines for trends, then adapt them to suit your features.

Lighten up. Heavy makeup is ageing. Try using fewer items, subtly blended. Making up in natural daylight stops you getting heavy-handed and improves your accuracy. Use daylight effect or hobby bulbs, which are recommended for artwork and other close work, for making up at night.

Heavy makeup is ageing

Brush up on technique. Buy some new applicators – they'll help you make quick, light, professional work of your new look. But don't forget fingers are natural blenders, too. They help makeup to look less contrived.

FOUNDATION – COMPLEXION BASICS

If you've never worn a base before, it might be time to consider it now. Foundations even out a patchy skintone and give a colour-boosting veil to pale complexions. But it's not their job to change your skintone – real 'second skin' tones (ie shades which genuinely look as natural as a second skin) vanish without tidemarks. Always test them in the store on your cheek, not your hands.

WHICH TEXTURES WORK BEST?

Heavy, creamy bases tend to sink into lines. Light, polymer-based fluids glide on smoothly and cling without clumping. Powder or cream compact formulas are easy to sponge on and give slightly more coverage without looking heavy. But avoid very matt, long-lasting or non-transfer formulas – they dry far too fast and can look heavy, dead or patchy. The most flattering textures contain light-reflective pigments that seem to even out shadows, furrows and texture problems, leaving skin looking smooth, dewy and alive – a huge plus for dry skins.

HOW TO APPLY THEM

Don't think you have to cover your entire face with foundation. Dot and blend a small amount where you really need to correct blotches and shadows, for example around the nose, over cheeks and chin and around the eyes. A scant blending over lids primes them for eyeshadow. Use your fingers to do the initial blending and a latex sponge to tidy up around crevices and hollows and prevent foundation clogging downy hairs on the face and hairline. A small, flat brush is ideal for sweeping out lines where too much base has gathered.

CONCEALER – HIDING WHAT YOU DON'T LIKE TO SEE

Concealer may be all you need to unify your skintone. American makeup artist Trish McEvoy uses hers instead of foundation to save time covering broken veins, spots and shadows around the nose, under the eyes and over the cheeks. Pick a shade that matches your base skintone exactly so that there are no obvious patches where you've tried to hide flaws.

> *Concealer may be all you need to unify your skintone*

WHICH TEXTURES WORK BEST?

Firm creams in stick or paste format give dense cover, but go lightly – they can sink into creases, especially around the eyes. Automatic fluids with sponge applicators are ideal for spot-checking and their slightly drier textures are often longer lasting.

HOW TO APPLY THEM

Print (rather than rub) on concealer using your fingertips, then blend it lightly with a soft, flat brush. This way, you won't rub or wipe it off again. Brushes also work better than fingers around curves and crevices and especially in inner eye corners.

POWDER – DO YOU NEED IT?

Not as much as you think. Since the introduction of polymers, makeup's stay-put agents, fluid textures are far more stable and less ready to move around on the face. Foundation only needs extra setting if your skin is oily or the area is highly mobile, like under eyes. On dry skin, too much powder can deaden a base's fresh, dewy finish. If you don't wear foundation, just concealer, a light overall dusting of powder unifies the skin with a 'dressed' but naturally smooth finish.

WHICH TEXTURES WORK BEST?

Choose an ultra-fine milled, translucent powder that won't change the colour of your base. If your skin is dry, look for a moisturizing formula. Slightly light-reflective powders avoid a matt, floury finish.

HOW TO APPLY THEM

Pick up a light coating on a velour puff and press over foundation or concealer. Lightly buff and flick off excess with a huge, soft complexion brush.

BLUSHER – YOUR VERY BEST ANTI-AGEING ALLY

'I always take my blushers everywhere I go,' says Bobbi Brown. 'They cheer me up because they give me a healthy look. I feel, and probably look, prettier.' Used prudently, blush is a girl's best friend. Putting selective colour back into your cheeks enlivens your entire face naturally and easily, without changing your base skintone. Get it right and you'll always look radiantly healthy.

WHICH TEXTURES WORK BEST?

Powders give a fine wash of colour, but some can look chalky or are too densely pigmented. Cream-to-powder pots and compacts with a very slight sheen look freshest, are most natural and are surprisingly easy to blend. Go for sandy-pink for fair skins; tawny-rose on medium skins; fresh rose on yellow-based skins and deep rose on dark skins. Bronzing powders make good blusher substitutes on all skin tones – choose pale, medium or dark according to your complexion. A shade that tones with your lipstick will always look the most meant to be.

Throw away stubby compact brushes

HOW TO APPLY THEM

Throw away stubby compact brushes.
Use a large, firm blusher brush for both powders and powder-creams, working them lightly into the base with a circular, polishing action. Use very little at first – it's far easier to build up than tone down. For an extra-natural look, Bobbi Brown layers a soft tone first, then adds a 'pop' of slightly brighter blush to highlight the cheekbone domes. Touch blusher over bronzing powder too, to stop it looking dingy. Where exactly do you blush? Bobbi Brown recommends you check your face after exercise or the shower, then echo the shade and shape where it flushes naturally. British-based makeup artist Ariane Poole gets her models to grin, then blushes the chubbed cheek apples. A touch on the chin, forehead and browbones gives an extremely healthy-looking, balancing flush.

EYESHADOWS – THE ENLIGHTENED TOUCH

Eyeshadows are often make or break factors on older faces. Deep shades make eyes look sunken, especially if lids are hooded; bright or pale tones emphasize dry lid creases. Forget complicated eye looks and concentrate on a single shade that gently defines and wakes up your eyes.

WHICH TEXTURES WORK BEST?

Again, powder-creams or very soft, velvety powders are easiest to blend and cover crinkly lids evenly. Avoid chalky matt textures that make lids look papery and pale shimmery shadows that highlight wrinkles. Compromise with very slightly sheeny shadows that open deep-set eyes without advertising lines and creases. Choose neutral shades like gentle browns or warm, sandy flesh tones.

Forget complicated eye looks

HOW TO APPLY THEM

If you're using powder shadow, dust closed lids with your translucent powder brush first. Then use a flat shadow brush to work colour over the lids smoothly, down into the lashline. If you're using a powder cream, touch it straight onto the centre lids with the sponge applicator, then blend with fingertips. Don't overdo it – colour should fade to nothing in the sockets and outer corners.

EYELINERS AND DEFINERS – SOFT OPTIONS, NO HARD EDGES

Defining eyes well is a hit-and-miss business. Instead of widening them, heavy lines 'close' eyes, giving them a hard look. But gentle definition gives shape to your eyes and depth to your lashes, especially if they're scanty.

WHICH TEXTURES WORK BEST?

Creamy pencils smudge into creases and it's difficult to paint a fine fluid line because it bumps along lid crinkles. The softest, most smudgeproof options are powder pencils or matt powder shadows chosen to blend with your lashes.

HOW TO APPLY THEM

Stroke pencils closest to the lash roots, from mid-lids to outer eye corners. Blend with a pointed latex applicator or very fine brush, blurring the line softly outwards. Use this technique with powder shadows, drawing the line first with the tip of your applicator. Defining the lower lashline only opens up eyes where the upper lid is so deepset that it's barely visible.

MASCARA – LASH LENGTHENERS OR BOOSTERS?

Lashes lose their length and volume with age but a good mascara puts back some of the natural definition, bringing eyes into focus again.

WHICH TEXTURES WORK BEST?

A couple of coats of a lash-lengthening formula are more likely to go on smoothly without clumping than a lash-building mascara. Avoid waterproof mascaras for regular use – they are difficult to build up and can make lashes look spiky.

HOW TO APPLY THEM

Look up when you brush both sets of lashes – you're less likely to blob. Leave 30 seconds between each coat, then separate lashes with a lash comb – it really is a good investment. Tidy any smudges with a damp cotton bud. If your lashes are stubby and you can't coat the bottom ones without blobbing, just leave them bare.

LIPSTICKS – WARM, LIVELY COLOUR

A soft, dewy mouth is your face's sexiest asset. Along with

blush, lip tint works hardest to put your face in focus – notice how all your features suddenly wake up when you slick your lipstick on.

WHICH TEXTURES WORK BEST?

Long-lasting matt formulas deaden lips and dry into ugly ridges. Rich creams and glosses feather into crease lines round the lip contour. Compromise with firm-textured demi-matt or translucent textures. The most wearable tones are browny-pinks, soft corals and rose tones that boost the natural colour of your lips without showing up when they start to wear off. Avoid blue-pinks, bright reds and frosty textures – they all make older mouths look hard. Browns are too dull and beige is too bland.

HOW TO APPLY THEM

Slick them straight from the bullet onto the centre of your lips, then use a brush to work in the colour firmly and tidy the contours. Blot on a tissue, then brush over again without reloading colour.

Tricks with light

Complexion primers add a wash of corrective colour to liven up dull skin, used alone or under foundation. Apply them sparingly, centralizing colour on cheeks, chin, nose and forehead.

- Green calms redness.
- Mauve lifts sallow, olive skin.
- Peach and pink warm pasty skin.
- Light-reflective gold, silver or opalescent skin finishes 'lift' furrows and shadows, softly highlight strong features and give foundation a fresh, dewy finish.

TROUBLESHOOTING TECHNIQUES

Hide lines and wrinkles. Brush and blend pink-based 'light-ning touch' highlighters into frown lines, nose to lip creases and chin.

Minimize heavy, droopy browbones. Buff lightly with blusher, sweeping colour up and out towards temples.

Hide over-flushed cheeks. Blend in concealer, then add just a hint of blusher high on the cheekbones to make the glow look planned.

Boost spiky lashes. Coat them with colourless lash primer first, then brown-black lengthening mascara. Reapply colour if you need to and give lashes a final comb-through.

Open tired eyes. Blend concealer over under-eye shadows and in inner eye corners. Coat lids with a neutral colour, then highlight the centre domes. Define the lower lashline only. Use a lash-curler after mascara – it really does leave eyes wide open.

Strengthen a weak lipline and flesh out a skinny mouth. Apply a conditioning lip fix formula to plump and firm skin, tighten crinkles and keep lipstick from feathering. Use a natural lip-toned pencil to draw in a smooth contour, then a lip brush to soften the edges and fill colour in over the lips. Top with toning lipstick, but don't go right to the edge. Blot with a tissue, then plump up lip centres only with a subtle sheeny gloss.

Grooming brows

Eyebrows give your face expression, so make sure it's a gentle, warm one. The ideal brow shape starts in line with the inner eye corner, arches gently upwards two-thirds of the way over the eye at the browbone peak, then tapers gently just beyond the outer eye corner.

- Thin out bushy brows that bear down on eyes. Pluck stragglers from the browbone and over the nose bridge. But go easy – overplucking gives you a shocked, hard look.
- Feather out skinny overplucked brows. Use a firm-textured sharp pencil matched to their shade, or a tone lighter. Best of all are powder pencils that look realistic and don't melt or shine as the day wears on. Sketch in hair-fine strokes, feathered to mimic natural hair.
- Fill in patchy brows with a powder pencil, or work in brown powder eyeshadow with a stiff wedge-shaped brush.
- If your brows are white or fair, consider having them tinted at a salon – but don't attempt this yourself.

TEN-MINUTE TIP

Fake a fresh, glowing face

This is the maximum impact, miminum effort 'healthy look' makeup that wins you compliments. Make it your second-nature daily basic – you really can do it all in time.

- Dot concealer over cheeks, chin, around nostrils, under eyes and on centre lids, then finger-blend. Two minutes.
- Stroke neutral brown automatic powder-cream shadow over lid centres then finger-blend all over lids. Two minutes.
- Lightly apply golden-bronze powder or powder-cream over cheek apples, browbones, chin and forehead. Two minutes.
- Brush a single coat of brown-black mascara on upper and

lower lids. Tidy up blobs underneath lashes with a barely damp cotton bud or clean sponge-tip shadow applicator. This will leave a faint shadow, as if you had just applied eye definer. Three minutes.

- Straight from the bullet, slick on rose, brown-pink or peach-toned translucent lipstick – shades with a slight goldlit sheen are lively and flattering. Use a lipbrush to tidy the edges if you need to. One minute.

TEN TIPS FOR A 'BAD FACE' DAY

- **Flash-fix your skin.** Use a 'morning after' moisturizer with a temporary tightening, brightening formula (like Clarin's classic Beauty Flash) to pep up and smooth a sad complexion.
- **Buff on bronzer.** A touch of powder whisked over cheek-bones, browbones and chin gives a pale face a healthy looking glow.
- **Go pink.** Avoid hard-to-wear reds and dull browns. Rose tones on lips and cheeks are easy-going, gentle flatterers that soften your look.
- **Try power-walking part way to work.** Get some oxygen into your bloodstream and the roses back into your cheeks. Pounding out stress and tension irons the lines smoother, too.
- **Slap-tap your face in the shower.** The rush of blood to your cheeks helps firm your face and leaves you looking like you've just sprinted ten miles.
- **Have sex.** Makeup artists say that the energy surge of sex in the morning plumps up skin and gives it the freshest kind of afterglow.
- **Freshen up dull, dry skin.** Soak a cotton wool pad in glycerine and rosewater (from chemists), then buff all over your face. Skin looks soft and dewy and makeup lasts longer.

- **Use a highlighter.** Bounce light off dark shadows and wake up tired eyes with pinky-gold shimmer powder on centre lids and inner eye corners.
- **Hide puffy eyes.** Use a slightly deeper shadow than normal to 'shrink back' swollen lids. Cream textures are gentlest.
- **Choose a shade brighter lipstick.** If your skin looks 'grey', a slightly richer lip tint enlivens your whole face, without you having to pile on extra makeup.

Polish performance

Don't think your nails have to match your lipstick. No-colour polishes which just add a blush and a sheen groom nails beautifully without showing chips. Subtly shimmery, opalescent pinks or flesh-toned tints are pretty and practical – a single coat gives a subtle sheen that suits and enlivens all hands and nails. Choose your nail shade to flatter your skintone.

- If your hands are pale, avoid blue-pinks, very pale silver and ivory, which will make them look cold.
- If your hands have brown patches, avoid beige tones and opt for warmer roses.
- Hands that tend to redness look cooler against silver-beige polish.
- Forget bright red and deep plum polishes – they're too stark and harsh to flatter older hands.

CHAPTER 6

Haircare
No more bad hair days!

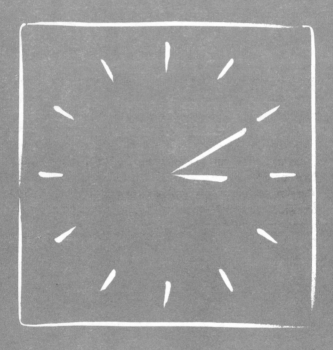

Your hair gets you noticed first. A good style can take years off your face in minutes: a bad one can drag your looks down. Experiment with warm colour and soft styling to make your hair your greatest ally.

WHICH STYLE FLATTERS YOUR FACE?

Avoid:
- **Straight, droopy styles.** They literally drag you down, emphasizing saggy features, such as a loose jaw and eyebags. On thin faces, they're deadly.
- **Scraped-back styles.** They're far too severe. Pulling hair back from the face exposes lines around your eyes and forehead, and 'blue' veins on your temples. They also leave your face looking gaunt.
- **Very long hair.** It's too high-maintenance, and frankly, a bit too girly. If you can't bear short hair, have yours trimmed to a bouncier shoulder or jaw length.

Go for:
- **Short, upbeat styles.** Cut well, they're like an instant face lift as all the attention is 'swept up'. Short hair is easier to care for, too, especially if it's tinted and the ends tend to go frizzy or dry.
- **Feather cuts and soft fringes.** Layers are your best allies. They allow you to fluff hair up and away from the scalp, creating fullness, while softening your hairline. If your hair's tinted, they also help you hide your roots. Fringes hide lined

foreheads and flatter the eye area. Loose-layered bobs look contemporary without being too girly, but keep them on the short side.

- **Neat, sleek bobs.** These look groomed and youthful. The best cuts – around jaw-length – make even fine hair look full and swingy. But avoid them if your hair is tinted – the inevitable parting advertises regrowth.

GETTING THE SHAPE YOU WANT

MOUSSES

These are the easiest body-builders to use, but some hair-dressers say they dull the hair, leaving a sticky or powdery residue. Keep quantities realistic – a golfball-sized dollop is enough for most short to jaw-length styles. Comb evenly through damp hair before styling.

GELS

As the firmest styling formulas, they can leave hair stiff. Again, don't overdo them. To perk up fine hair without weighing down the tips, concentrate the gel at the roots, massaging it in place with your fingertips, then combing through so the ends get the least. Apply to damp hair before blow-drying or styling.

GLOSSING SERUMS

These shine and tame dull, frizzy hair and add extra polish to coloured hair. Use them very sparingly – a single drop may be enough for a whole head of hair. Spread serum in the palms of your hands and massage through dry hair after styling, or massage into the ends only to 'mend' splits. Fine spray glossers are easy to use and less likely to overload hair.

POMADES, WAXES, PUTTIES AND STYLING CREAMS

These are specialist finishing formulas which mould the hair into place, giving texture and sheen. Pomades give a high-shine finish, waxes a more subtle polish. Stiffer putties and styling creams coax hair sections into soft peaks or ruffle them into highly textured looks. Professional stylists say they give baby-soft hair the same kind of manageable grip as 'day old' hair after washing. Massage all these formulas sparingly through dry hair.

FINISHING SPRAYS

Use these to fix the style and hold the lift. Misted onto damp hair, they also help mould blow-dry or roller styles. Choose regular, firm or extra-firm hold according to your hair's flop factor. Aim the spray towards the roots, and avoid 'rock solid' looks. Hair flatters most when it's just less than perfect. Allow it to move – a little.

> *Hair flatters most when it's just less than perfect*

HAIR LOSS

It's natural to lose 40–60 hairs each day, but over 100 is a worry. Human hair goes through 'moult' phases – you may notice more stray hairs in the sink or brush in spring and autumn. In women, oestrogen governs hair growth, preventing it from growing on the face and diverting it to the head, which is why women tend to have more lustrous hair than men. But when oestrogen levels drop at the menopause, hair becomes noticeably thinner. The actual diameter of individual head hairs also begins to decrease as early as 25, accounting for a gradual loss in 'body'. As a final insult, some women may begin to lose their hair altogether. What hastens the loss?

Hair growth slows with age. The wind-down begins in our thirties and by the fifties, our active hair follicles have virtually halved. Stress is a significant factor: even in women, it triggers androgenic (male) hormones also responsible for male pattern baldness. Neck and shoulder tension also restricts circulation to the scalp, and follicles may become weak and malnourished. Similarly, strict diets, periods of illness or medical treatments like chemotherapy and radiotherapy may cause hair to fall.

Rough handling causes casualties. Black women have the highest rate of traction hair loss, due to tugging at tangles. Harsh straightening chemicals also encourage hair to snap at its weak points. Chemical abuse – over-perming and colouring – is also the most common cause of Caucasian hair damage. Sleeping in too-tight rollers stresses the scalp and can cause clumpy hair loss.

To limit losses, avoid rough brushing and heat styling. Use mild, non-detergent shampoos, massaging the scalp gently. Sadly, no cosmetic formula has been ultimately clinically proven to stimulate hair growth or significantly prevent loss. Recently, however, l'Oréal launched a promising massage system under their Kerastase label. Vials of an 'active' fluid contain a plant-based molecule that prevents collagen at the roots from hardening and starving hair growth. Trials at Amersham Hospital in the UK suggested a 5 per cent loss reduction in six weeks.

GREY HAIR

Hair gets its colour from granules of melanin pigment produced by cells in the hair follicle. As we get older, these melanocyte cells become less active and grey hairs start to appear. Hair turns totally white when the melanocytes cease to function altogether, but why is still a mystery. Here, though, are some grey hair facts.

Large doses of B vitamins can reverse greying in three months

- Most Caucasian women start to go grey at 30 and by 50 at least half their head will be grey. Black people go grey more slowly, sometimes as late as their mid-forties; Japanese and Asian women start greying in their late thirties. Dark-haired people are thought to go grey faster, but this is just because the 'rogue' hairs are more obvious.
- It's a myth that grey hair is coarser than pigmented hair, but pulling out grey hairs distorts the follicle and crinkly hairs grow back.
- Nutrition and stress also affect hair colour. Stress burns up B vitamins in the body, and so does alcohol. A diet insufficient in these vitamins may also hasten the appearance of grey hairs. According to trichologist Philip Kingsley, studies have shown that large doses of B vitamins can reverse greying in three months; but stop the vitamins and the grey starts again.
- To go grey gradually, see hints on colour, page 78.

BEATING DANDRUFF

Stress, hormonal changes and too much sugar and salt in the diet can influence the scalp's sweat and sebum output. Bacteria on the scalp cause surface cells to shed and stick together in oily clumps, yet hair tips can seem dry and coarse. Here's Philip Kingsley's solution to controlling grease at the roots and relieving dry hair.

- Alternate your regular shampoo with an anti-dandruff formula, and condition the hair tips only.
- Rinse thoroughly after cleansing to keep scurf at bay. Surfactants from shampoos can irritate and dry the scalp, and turn to dandruff-like powder if left in the hair.
- Use a clarifying shampoo every three or four washes to remove residues from body-building shampoo and styling products.

Left unchecked, dandruff can cause hair loss. If your scalp becomes excessively scaly, sore or itchy, see a trichologist or dermatologist.

CAN YOU SHAMPOO THE LIFE BACK INTO YOUR HAIR?

Shampooing is the make or break factor of hair health. But does frequent washing harm hair? Not necessarily, says trichologist Philip Kingsley, who recommends daily shampooing with a mild formula to cleanse and stimulate the scalp and flush away loose strands that may matt and tangle the hair. But these days, a shampoo's brief goes beyond cleansing – it's expected to treat your hair problems too. So which formula should you choose?

REGULAR USE, PH-BALANCED

Non-alkaline, detergent-free, acid-balanced shampoos help prevent dryness and scalp irritation. Joan Newton, Training Manager at Redken UK, explains that daily washing with alkaline shampoos means that scalp oils have little chance to coat hair thoroughly. Greasy scalps also benefit from regular mild treatment, as alkaline stripping causes increased oil production. The milder your shampoo, the smoother and glossier your hair will be. With a pH of 7, water alone can swell hair, ruffling up its cuticles so it loses its smooth compactness. Bacteria thrive on a pH of around 6.8, so over-washing may also encourage scalp infections. A shampoo with a pH of between 4.5 and 5.5 pulls the hair together and maintains the scalp's equilibrium. Professional tinters also recommend pH-balanced shampoos to help keep the hair cuticle tight and the colour in the hair.

CONDITIONING SHAMPOOS

The cleansing agents in these shampoos leave the hair shaft with a negative charge. Positive ions in the moisturizing ingredients cling to the negatively charged hair shafts to help eliminate static and prevent frizziness, flyaway and tangling. These can be useful formulas if your hair is coarse, brittle, dry or coloured. But be warned: hairdressers hate combined 2-in-1 formulas because of the build-up – even shampoo-soluble silicones in these formulas can be difficult to get rid of. Heat styling bakes them in and the hair goes limp, warns Redken's Joan Newton. Philip Kingsley agrees. Shampoo first, condition after, he advises.

> *Hairdressers hate combining 2-in-1 formulas because of the build-up*

CLARIFYING SHAMPOOS

A build-up of sticky styling products and body-building ingredients magnetizes grime that progressively weakens hair, weighs it down and makes it dull and difficult to style. Some clingy ingredients also block perming and colouring agents, so results are unpredictable. Clarifying shampoos are 'detox' treatments that use chelating ingredients to break the bonds of polymers and mineral deposits so that they can be neutralized and flushed away. Some formulas also neutralize swimming pool chlorine, which fades tinted hair. But some hairdressers warn that clarifying shampoos can also leach out professional colour, too, so don't overuse them – every sixth wash should do.

KEEPING HAIR IN POLISHED CONDITION

Conditioners are anti-ageing creams for hair. They build in moisture and gloss by smoothing hair cuticles, preventing tangles and buffering hair against heat styling and environmental hazards such as ultraviolet damage and frizz-causing, humid air. Choose the right conditioner for your hair type. Dry hair needs intensive moisture formulas. Coarse, curly, brittle hair may benefit from leave-in conditioners, massaged into the tips. Coloured and permed hair needs moisturing proteins and UV-filters to compensate for chemical damage and prevent colour fade. Fine, lank or greasy hair needs lightweight formulas – conditioning sprays and mousses often work well. Whichever the formula, don't overdo it. A 50p-sized blob should service most heads of hair. How long should you leave a rinse-off conditioner? Some experts say a full three minutes – longer if your hair is extra-dry. Others say it hardly matters – you can rinse it off almost immediately. The most important thing is to make sure each strand is evenly coated first. (See washing tips on page 77).

> *Conditioners are anti-ageing creams for hair*

DO INTENSIVE PACKS DO ANY GOOD?

According to the research and development department at Alberto V05, special care formulas contain more active ingredients than regular conditioners. Some penetrate the hair, but their main job is to smooth damaged cuticles and leave a light-reflective shine. How long their effects last depends on how porous your hair is, but intensive conditioners generally do last longer because they're more difficult to wash out than regular formulas. According to Philip Kingsley, clingy ingredients like silicones and oils can linger for up to a week – not always what fine, floppy hair really needs. The maxim here is don't overdo it. But rather than risk going limp under heavy, post-shampoo packs, Kingsley advocates using pre-shampoo treatments that plump up the hair's moisture quota, then shampooing them out, leaving just enough conditioner to 'fill in the cracks'. A pre-shampoo treatment with a conditioning oil (olive and sunflower oil work as well as commercial 'hot oil' treatments) also softens dry weak hair and prevents the shampoo over-stripping moisture.

DO HAIR THICKENERS WORK?

The haircare industry estimates that 70 per cent of British women believe that their hair is so fine it needs building up. Hair thickeners rely on substantive ingredients, which cling to individual hair shafts and build up over several treatments. Spray-on lotions and volumizing shampoos and conditioners invariably contain a cocktail of resins, plant proteins or keratin, the hair's own protein. According to Wella, whose Liquid Hair formula pioneered the hair-thickening market, keratin molecules act as building blocks, repairing and rebuilding the hair's internal structure. Vitamin B5 (d-panthenol) and plant proteins such as wheatgerm and soy also help to nourish and strengthen. The only problem is that too much ingredient build-up makes hair either stiff or floppy. The worst culprits of all are silicones, which need thoroughly removing with a 'detox' shampoo at least once a week.

BRUSHING IN GLOSS

Brushing 'dusts' your hair, clearing it of stray hairs, stale scalp cells and styling products. Hairdressers suggest we should brush thoroughly before each shampoo, as a pre-cleanse stage. A brush last thing at night loosens mousse, gels and sprays and relaxes the scalp, while brushing first thing in the morning lifts flattened hair from the scalp. Avoid sharp-bristled brushes which scratch the scalp and split hairs. Rubber-cushioned designs with well-spaced, flexible bristles are gentlest. The longer your hair, the larger your brush should be: the thicker your hair, the denser the brush bristles. Some experts believe natural bristles absorb more sebum and are better 'cleansers', but make sure they're round-tipped. Don't over-brush – it can weaken fragile hair. A hundred strokes is far too many. As for combs, antistatic hard rubber or vulcanite models with saw-cut, individually smoothed teeth are the professional choice. Wide teeth distribute conditioner without stressing wet hair. Tail combs are handy for sectioning off hair prior to blow-drying. Use a comb to untangle the hair, working from the tips to the roots, progressively smoothing snags with a light, upwards flicking movement. Never tug.

> *Natural bristles absorb more serum and are better 'cleansers'*

Wash day dos

- Gently does it – and don't overdo it. A good shampoo cleanses hair thoroughly without tangling or stressing the roots.
- Use a wide-toothed comb to untangle dry hair and prevent matting once it's wet.
- Thoroughly wet hair needs less shampoo. Use warm water and gently comb your fingers through the hair to ensure it's really soaking.
- Rub shampoo in the palms of your hands, then smooth over your hair. Use your palms to distribute suds and your finger-tips to gently knead your scalp. Massage for around three minutes, untangling your hair from front to back every so often with your fingers.
- Use clear, running warm water – not hot – and don't skimp. A common cause of dull hair is insufficient rinsing – keep going even when you think your hair is clean. If you can stand it, finish with a cold jet to tone the scalp and close the hair cuticles.
- Smooth conditioner over your hair with the palms of your hands, concentrating on the ends and avoiding the scalp. Rinse thoroughly again.
- Wrap your hair in a towel and squeeze out the excess water. Untangle with a wide-toothed comb, starting from the ends. Now you're ready to style.

TEN-MINUTE TIP

Relaxing scalp massage

Massage boosts the scalp's circulation, increasing nutrient supply to the roots. It may also help to prevent hair loss. Be gentle, though – vigorous massage can irritate the scalp and loosen weak roots.

- Brush your hair first to make sure it won't tangle.
- Start by kneading your shoulders to ease tension there, then work upwards over your neck. Remember, a stiff neck leads to a tense scalp.
- Ease your fingertips under the bulk of your hair and massage gently around the roots, using kneading and subtle vibration movements.
- Cover the entire scalp, working from the base of the skull to the crown, from the brow to the crown and from the sides to the crown. Finish by gently massaging the temples.

HOME COLOUR KNOW-HOW

Home colour used to be a hit and miss business, but technology has moved on since the days of horror stories about green hair. The new-generation home 'hair cosmetic' formulas are easy to use and colour-accurate – so long as you do as you're told. Colour expert Jo Hansford, who now has her own home colour range, advises you read the instructions at least three times to make sure you get every stage right. If you're a colour virgin, she adds, choose your ideal colour by staying within two or three shades either way of your natural tone. Her favourite formulas are demi-permanents that don't change or lighten hair but enrich it with warm, glossy overtones. You can also use demis to blend in first grey hair, refresh tired permanent colour and perk up or calm down highlights. If you're going seriously grey and considering permanent colour, it may be a mistake, says Jo, to try to re-create your original colour. As the skin pales with age, a dark tone may be too harsh now. Blonde, on the other hand, can look washed out. Rich light browns with a hint of chestnut suit a broad range of complexions and give the skin the warmth and liveliness it needs now.

PERMANENT COLOUR

This covers grey completely, lightens or darkens hair and lasts until it grows out. An alkaline agent (usually ammonia) swells the hair and opens the outer cuticle so pigment molecules can enter the hair shaft. An oxidizing agent such as hydrogen peroxide lightens the hair's natural pigment and causes the pigment molecules to produce the larger molecules that create its new colour.

TONE-ON-TONE TINTS

Also called demi-permanents, these formulas cover up to 60 per cent grey and last around 20 washes. They colour the hair to the same depth, or deeper. The ammonia-free and low alkaline and oxidizing formula mean tone-on-tones can't lighten or significantly alter natural colour, but they're excellent for enriching and enlivening hair and are ideal first-time tints.

SEMI-PERMANENT TINTS

These 'shampoo-in' formulas cover up to 40 per cent grey and enrich and deepen your hair colour but won't lighten it. The colour washes out over eight or so shampoos as pigment molecules lodge in the outer layers of the hair cortex only. Semis are the most user-friendly colourants – if the colour's not quite right, you're not stuck with it. You can also use them to tone down or refresh tired highlights.

PROFESSIONAL TIPS FOR TROUBLEPROOF TINTING

- Your natural hair colour and its condition influence the results of a tint. Always run a test on a tiny section first before you do your whole head. Then follow the instructions to the letter.
- Tint in the kitchen, not the bathroom, to avoid splashing and staining carpets and loo seats. If you have a mixer tap, you can rinse over the kitchen sink much more easily than over the bath. Cover the floor with paper to protect porous tiles.
- Protect yourself with a black bin liner, making holes for your head and arms. It's much simpler than fiddling with plastic capes or towels.
- Prevent the tint from staining your skin by blocking your hairline and ears with petroleum jelly, but make sure it doesn't touch your hair.
- Colour can get runny when your head is warm. Pin a cotton-wool sausage around your hairline and the edge of the plastic cap included in the package to catch any drips.
- If colour does stain your skin, massage gently with your regular facial exfoliator.
- Once you've applied the tint, five minutes of gentle hairdryer heat encourages it to bond and gives deeper, richer colour, especially on grey hair.
- Protect your new colour and help it to last with special formula colour-saving shampoos and conditioners.

HOW ABOUT HIGHLIGHTS?

Natural hair is made up of several depths of tone that add to its texture and gloss, which is why 'block' or single-tone colour never looks completely convincing. Highlights and lowlights that combine two, three or more tints mimic natural hair highs and lows. They don't have to be blonde – a couple of shades lighter around the hairline, merging with warmer tones over the crown, can subtly brighten your features. Best of all, highlights blend in with grey, camouflaging rather than covering. But in all honesty, it's virtually impossible to do highlights at home. Best visit a salon.

Hair mascaras – magic wands?

If you thought they were kid's stuff, think again. In among the techno blues and fuschias, some cosmetic companies offer softer coppery, sandy and ebony shades that come in pretty useful for retouching roots or slicking out sprinklings of grey. They're strictly wash-out remedies, but they'll tide you over until your next retint.

A WORD ON PERMS

Tight, frizzy curls are outdated, ageing and damaging. Like permanent colour, perms roughen and dry hair cuticles, especially if they're set on small curling rods. If your hair needs 'oomph', a body wave with a gentler, less alkaline solution may be the answer. Aimed at the roots, these waves 'lift' fine, limp hair from the scalp without damaging vulnerable tips and work best where hair is layered but still tends to flop.

HEAT STYLING HOW-TO

Heat-styling damages and frazzles hair like nothing else. Forget curling tongs – it's too easy to singe both your hair and scalp. But used wisely, your hairdryer is your greatest style ally. Follow these steps to blow-drying your hair successfully without drying it out.

- Shampoo, condition and blot excess moisture with a towel. Apply styling product.
- To minimize heat intensity, your hair should be 50 per cent dry before you start precision blow-drying. Either leave it to dry naturally or rough-dry it with a cool hairdryer.
- For smooth styles, blow dry your hair in sections. Pin the top sections out of the way and dry the underneath sections first. Coax the hair around a large round brush, rotating it as you slowly and firmly pull it through the hair from roots to tips.
- For more textured styles, use the fingers of your free hand. Making a spider-shape with your fingers and gently massaging the roots lifts them away from the scalp and builds in texture. 'Scissoring' sections of hair from roots to tips between your fingers styles it more smoothly. When your hair is barely damp, light, circular massage with your palm will give an incredible lift.
- Keep the dryer on medium heat and about 10–15cm (4–6 inches) away from your hair. Aim the nozzle down the hair shafts from roots to tips. This flattens the cuticles, so that they reflect the light more and the hair looks glossy. Once the hair is dry, a final blast with the cold setting hardens and seals the cuticles in place.
- Use the right attachment for the job. The nozzle of your hairdryer concentrates hot air for quick, sleek, precision styling. The diffuser distributes warm air over a wider area and is ideal for initial 'rough' drying or styling naturally curly or wavy hair.

TEN-MINUTE TIP

Roller-boost flat hair
Velcro rollers are fast workers – they grip the hair smoothly and stay firm without pins. Choose large sizes to root-lift longer hair; smaller ones to build bounce into short hair. This tip works well as a boost between shampoos.

- Comb just-damp hair into sections and roll into rollers, lifting hair away from the scalp as you go.
- When your whole head is set, mist with hairspray.
- Blast with a hairdryer for five minutes.
- When your hair is dry, slide out the rollers and brush gently smooth. Alternatively, scrunch with your fingers for a soft, textured look.

CHAPTER 7

Bodycare
Maintaining the
superstructure

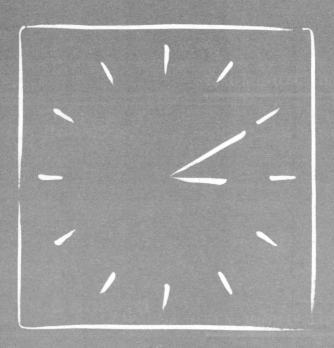

Get a grip on gravity. Look as good out of your clothes as you do in them, with this top-to-toe guide to staying firm, flexible, smooth and sensual.

TONING THE ZONES

NECK

Lines and slackness here are obviously ageing and hard to hide. Neck skin is thinner and drier than that on the face, with fewer naturally protective sebaceous glands to guard against moisture loss. Soaps, detergents and perfumes all dehydrate and sensitize the neck to other irritants such as scratchy roll necks, scarves and extremes of environmental temperature.

- Cleanse gently. Use a mild exfoliator to disperse sub-skin spots and rough patches. Then tone with an alcohol-free toner like rosewater, sweeping firmly upwards with a saturated cotton pad.
- Moisturize thoroughly but lightly. Serums and light lotions sink in fast and don't rub off on clothes or attract grime from the atmosphere. If your skin can tolerate them, vitamin A creams help smooth and prevent crêpey 'turkey neck' skin. A sunscreen is vital – check there's one in your moisturizer formula or top your moisturizer with an SPF15 lotion. Don't forget that the back of your neck is especially vulnerable to sun damage if your hair is short.

CHEST

The skin is still thin but is oilier than that of the neck, thanks to a denser concentration of oil glands. But sun damage shows as V-shaped creases, and crinkly, crêpey skin around the cleavage zone.

- Vitamin A creams help refine furrows and crinkles. Once again, a good sunscreen is vital, especially if you want to keep your plunging necklines.
- Avoid spraying perfumes on your chest and neck. Psoralins in some citrus scents are photosensitizers that magnify UV rays on skin. The result can be dingy-looking brown patches on the neck and chest, which are also encouraged by hormones in some brands of the Pill and HRT. Always spray scent where the sun can't get at it.

> *Always spray scent where the sun can't get at it*

TEN-MINUTE TIP

Neck and chest tonic
Follow this routine each time you apply body lotion or throat cream.

- Using the backs of both hands alternately, lightly stroke from your chest up the front of your neck, under your chin and over your jawline. Do at least ten strokes with each hand.
- Quickly and lightly slap under your chin with the back of one hand 30 times.
- Using one hand, place your fingertips on one side of your throat and your thumb on the other. Make firm and rapid

but gentle circular movements up and down your throat five times. Repeat with the other hand.

BREASTS

The breasts are supported by the Cooper's ligaments, which run from the nipples to their outer edges. Their only relevant muscles – the pectorals – run from the outsides of the upper breasts to the armpits, suspending the considerable weight of their soft adipose fatty tissue. With age and breast-feeding the breasts may become pendulous, taxing ligaments and muscles and stretching the skin. After the menopause, when body fat begins to diminish, the breasts lose weight and begin to take on a flatter, more hollow appearance. When skin loses its elasticity, breasts sag too. Is there anything you can do that a balcony bra can't?

- Bust creams can't firm or lift, but they do help to keep skin supple, smooth and toned. Splash breasts with cold water before you stroke on a cream for an extra tonic effect.
- Regular stroking massage also helps you check for lumps, but don't knead, prod or press too deeply.
- Once a week, gently exfoliate the breasts by lightly dry brushing or use a body scrub. AHA lotions also help to maintain surface smoothness.
- Get a good bra. You should comfortably fill the cups without spilling out at the sides or heaving over the tops. The under-band, sides and back should be firm, without digging in. Your breasts should be lifted up and away from your ribs – underwired cups are the most supportive. Wear your bra during the day, especially for exercising, but never in bed. According to American researchers Sydney Singer and Soma Grismijer, wearing a bra for more than 12 hours a day can increase the risk of breast cancer by 11 per cent. Bras

can constrict lymphatic points, encouraging toxic build-up and precipitating tumours, they argue.

TEN-MINUTE TIP

Bust boosters
Isometric presses help to raise the profile of the breasts by toning the pectoral (chest) muscles directly above them. Whether you do them sitting or standing, keep your back straight.

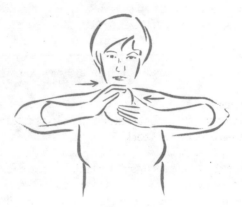

- Raise your elbows out to shoulder level and hold a ball about 10cm (4 inches) in front of you. Squeeze as hard as you can for a count of five.
- Bring your elbows together in front of you and hold the ball just above your head. Squeeze and hold for a count of five.
- Bring your elbows out to the side again and raise the ball over the crown of your head. Squeeze and hold.
- Push the ball straight out in front of you and, keeping your arms at shoulder height, squeeze and hold.

STOMACH

A 'bit of a tummy' is most women's least favourite feminine attribute. By the time we're 40, few of us have flat, taut tummies, especially if we've had children. But we can help keep the skin smooth and the muscles controlled.

- Moisturizing with vitamin A and AHA-based creams may help minimize stretch marks. Avoid rapid weight gains and losses, too.
- Exercise tones slack muscles and streamlines your body profile. As stomach muscles help to support the lower back, keeping them tuned helps avoid back pain.

TEN-MINUTE TIP

Tummy crunches
This exercise works your stomach muscles and helps strengthen a weak lower back.

- On your back, legs bent, feet hip-width, rest your hands on your thighs.
- Pull your stomach muscles in towards the floor. Slide your hands to your knees as you curl your body upwards and raise your head and shoulders off the floor. Hold for a count of five, then relax to a count of five.
- Repeat 10–25 times.

TEN-MINUTE TIP

Look like you've lost 3.2kg (7lb) in ten minutes
Good posture pulls your stomach in and makes you look instantly taller, slimmer and more elegant. Repeat this

realignment exercise at least three times a day so that good posture becomes second nature.

- Stand against a wall, knees relaxed and feet hip-width apart about 30cm (12 inches) away from the wall. Pull your stomach muscles towards the wall. Breathe out and press your head, shoulders, upper back and hips into the wall.
- Keep your spine straight and stomach muscles taut. Push away from the wall with your hands into a freestanding position. Look straight ahead without raising or jutting your chin. Relax your shoulders without slouching.

LEGS

You like to show them off – but what shape are they in? A sedentary lifestyle causes most of the age-related problems legs endure. Spending long periods sitting down leads to stiff joints, restricted circulation, puffy ankles and problems with veins. The best advice is to get out of the chair – and get walking!

- Spider or thread veins (telangiectasia) often appear on the thighs and the inside of the knees. They are capillaries with weakened, dilated walls and may be genetically inherited or induced by long-term use of steroids, pregnancy or severe overweight. Vitamin K creams help 'heal' leaky capillaries. The clinical treatment is sclerotherapy, where an inflammatory fluid is injected into the capillaries to seal them off. Lasers are also used to vaporize capillaries. Meantime, hide them with waterproof, heavy-duty camouflage cream, like Dermablend.

- Varicose veins which appear from mid-life onwards are becoming increasingly common. The causes are a low-fibre diet and a sedentary lifestyle, both of which lead to constipation, overweight and increased pressure on the legs. Pregnancy also triggers them, partly due to the sheer weight the legs are required to carry but also as a result of hormonal changes which relax and dilate the vein walls to accommodate the 50 per cent increase of blood in the body.

Varicose veins are ugly and painful; they throb, ache, and cause night cramps and swollen ankles in hot weather and during menstruation and long periods of standing. Walking, which gets the blood pumping through, temporarily relieves the discomfort. Treatment

Exercising and swimming help to prevent varicose veins

may be sclerotherapy, but the recurrence rate after ten years is as high as 90 per cent. The more permanent solution is surgery. Exercising and swimming help to prevent varicose veins. Avoid sitting with your legs crossed or pressing on a hard chair edge. Put your feet up at regular intervals during the day and especially in the evening. Eat a fibre-rich diet to prevent constipation. Supplements containing silica strengthen vein walls; and gingko biloba boosts circulation.

- Puffy, end-of-day ankles get worse as we get older. If your ankles become very puffy and the skin is taut and shiny, check with your doctor that the problem is not liver, kidneys or heart-related. A sedentary lifestyle, excess weight, pregnancy and some types of the Pill also cause swollen ankles by encouraging veins to dilate and become less efficient at draining excess fluid. Exercise – especially stairwalking and cycling – certainly helps. Support tights with graduated compression from foot to thigh work like a passive massage to pump blood and lymph back up the legs to minimize swelling and take the weight off varicose veins. Cooling aromatherapy gels and sprays – especially if they contain peppermint – are a stimulating, on-the-spot tonic for jetlagged or hard-working legs. At the end of the day, reduce swelling fast by soaking legs up to the knees in alternate buckets of cold and lukewarm water to get the circulation going.

TEN-MINUTE TIP

Light leg massage
To firm skin and boost circulation, do this massage each time you apply body lotion.

- Sit on the floor, legs out in front of you. Bend the knee of each leg as you massage it, keeping the foot flat on the floor. With hands either side of your leg, stroke smoothly and firmly upwards from ankles to tops of thighs. Repeat five times on both legs.
- With alternate hands, knead each thigh, rhythmically squeezing and releasing. Then stroke upwards several times from the knee, one hand following the other.
- Knead your calf muscle with both hands, gently lifting and squeezing it away from the bone. Then stroke gently up the back of the leg.

HIPS AND THIGHS

Curvy hips are sexy. Lumpy hips and dimpled thighs are equally feminine, but a good deal less alluring. Sceptical medics say cellulite is just plain fat – so how come men don't get it? In the 1970s, research by Berlin doctors found that female fat cells are different: whereas men's fall into a compact, honeycomb pattern, women's stand in arch-shaped chambers. Under pressure, these chambers push up into the skin's surface, giving a puckered appearance. Gain weight and fat cells swell, stretching surface skin tightly over the lumps. Why? Blame it on hormones. Whereas testosterone shrinks fat cells in the lower male body, oestrogen pads out female hips, buttocks, thighs, even knees. Since oestrogen is also stored in fat, excess padding is not only linked to our monthly cycle, but protects the 'birthing zone' and provides extra energy reserves. Puberty, pregnancy, and the Pill all trigger cellulite. It may dwindle along with oestrogen levels at the menopause, but HRT can perpetuate it. How can we help to disperse it?

- Don't pummel. New thinking says it damages and weakens skin rather than breaking down fat. Gentle massage encourages normal circulation and aids the penetration of cellulite creams.
- Dry brush your skin. A contributory factor to spongy cellulite is the build-up of toxic fluids trapped between fat cells. Help boost lymphatic drainage with a soft but firm natural bristle brush, sweeping upwards from the soles of the feet, over thighs, hips and buttocks. Brush daily for tough cellulite or three or four times weekly to keep skin smooth. Shower afterwards, using cool jets as a massage tonic.

> *Brush daily for tough cellulite or three or four times weekly to keep skin smooth*

- Don't over-exercise. Stress and a sedentary lifestyle encourage cellulite, but muscle-building workouts worsen surface dimples by pushing granular fat cells up into the skin. Energy burners and circulation boosters such as power walking, cycling, step aerobics, skipping and rebounding all help.

Do thigh creams work?
Cellulite creams are designed to have a triple action. They

contain diuretics such as horse chestnut, ivy, butcher's broom and seaweed to aid lymphatic drainage; xanthines – caffeine derivatives such aminophylline, theophylline and kola – to boost fat burn-up and inhibit its storage; and, as it's also thought that cellulite is an age problem affecting weakened skin, strengthening ingredients to help reinforce inner resistance and improve surface smoothness so dimples are less likely to show. Antioxidants such as vitamins C and E inhibit free radicals, so help to preserve collagen, elastin and skin firmness. Vitamin A palmitate boosts collagen production. AHAs smooth the skin surface and may also encourage collagen production deeper down. But it's wise not to believe in miracles. Remember that cellulite is basically a hormonal problem. Cosmetic creams can't 'melt' fat significantly – only drugs can do that. Moisturizing and conditioning the skin's surface certainly helps, but your real key to success is a diet that discourages fatty build-up in the first place.

The thinner thighs diet
Foods that are easy to digest and metabolize are the key to a high-energy diet that won't go straight to your thighs.

- Eat plenty of fresh fruit and vegetables, steamed or raw for maximum nutrition. Well-cooked pulses such as lentils, mung beans and red kidney beans are good sources of fibre, which aids waste elimination.
- Be picky with proteins. Avoid hard-to-digest red meat and opt instead for lighter, white meats such as chicken and fish. Restrict or avoid dairy foods and eggs.
- Avoid sugars and starches, including biscuits, cakes, pastries, sweets and chocolate.
- Don't over-flavour foods. Limit salt, sugar and spices. Substitute fresh herbs and seeds.
- Avoid animal fats such as butter and restrict vegetable oils and spreads. Never, ever fry.

- Drink 1.5–2 litres ($2^1/_2$–$3^1/_2$ pints) of still water daily. Try to avoid coffee, tea, fizzy drinks and alcohol. Choose caffeine-free herb teas that encourage digestion.
- Don't smoke – it severely restricts circulation and ages skin.

TEN-MINUTE TIP

Fake a smooth, firm skin
Use sheeny highlights and contouring powders to cheat your best assets into shape.

- Deflect light away from dull, dimpled skin and create a smooth-looking surface. Add just a pinch of loose gold or silver shimmer powder to your regular body lotion and smooth over arms, thighs and shins.
- Tanned limbs look leaner, firmer. Get the effect without risking your skin – use a self-tanning formula, or mix bronzing powder with your body lotion.

HANDS

Because they're constantly exposed, signs of age are hard to hide. Don't let them give the game away.

- UV damage causes skin slackness, loss of tone and age spots. Protect hands with a handcream with an SPF15 sunscreen. Some formulas also contain skin-lightening ingredients such as liquorice and lemon. For stubborn age spots, try a 2 per cent hydroquinone cream which breaks down pigment just below the skin's surface.
- Dehydration ages hands fast and causes roughness and flaking. Always wear rubber gloves to protect them from household detergents. Lightweight surgical latex gloves

(from chemists) protect from grime and are ideal for dry housework and wearing under gardening gloves. In the winter, gloves also protect against dryness and chapping.

- Exfoliate to keep hands smooth. Once or twice weekly, use facial cleansing grains to work around the knuckles and over the backs of the hands to remove stains and rough dead skin. Rinse, dry thoroughly and moisturize well. AHA-based handcreams help minimize rough skin build-up and tough cuticles.

- Rescue severely dry, chapped hands with an overnight pack. Last thing at night, work a rich handcream into your hands, then work in a light layer of petroleum jelly. Sleep in cotton gloves to keep the pack on your hands and off the sheets.

- Nails like the sun – it stimulates their growth. But they also need to maintain at least 12 per cent moisture content to stay strong and flexible. Dehydration is a key cause of peeling, split and brittle nails. A good conditioning handcream will improve your nails too – massage it well around the nail base each time you apply, especially in cold, very dry weather.

- Nails age too. After 40, slower cell turnover means they tend to become more horny and ridged. Gently buff the surface smooth with an extra-fine emery board, then polish with a chamois buffer. Ridge-filling bases also help even the nail surface before you apply laquer.

TEN-MINUTE TIP

Flexy hand workout

This keeps wrists, hands, fingers and nails supple by boosting circulation and joint flexibility. Good circulation encourages nail growth, too. Do this quick routine each time you apply handcream.

- Hold one hand between the thumb and fingers of the other. With the thumb, massage between and along each finger with firm, circular movements. Then bend the first two fingers of one hand and grip the straight fingers of the other hand scissor-fashion, one at a time, gently pulling from base to tip.
- Massage the palm with the thumb, using firm circular movements. Now stroke upwards several times from palm to elbow. Finally massage around your wrist. Change hands.
- Rotate each finger gently three times in each direction. Now rotate the wrists. Gently bend each wrist backwards by pushing the heel of your other hand against the palm.
- Finish by letting your arms hang loosely by your sides, relaxing your hands, wrists and fingers.

Finger food

Strong, healthy nail growth relies on a good diet. The following nutrients are especially significant.

- Keratin – the tough, horny protein that forms nails – contains high levels of sulphur and selenium and moderately high levels of calcium, potassium and trace minerals.
- Iron and zinc deficiencies cause brittleness, as might a lack of sulphurous amino acids, vitamin B1 (thiamine) and vitamin C.
- Tests on smokers' nail clippings reveal low concentrations of all the vital minerals – possibly because smoking inhibits circulation.
- Research shows that the trace mineral silica strengthens the cross-links that bond keratin layers together, so helping to prevent splitting and flaking.
- It's a myth that gelatine strengthens nails. Likewise, white spots are more likely to be caused by damage to the base – the only living part of the nail – than a lack of calcium.

Cheat's manicure

This is your low-maintenance guide to well-groomed nails and younger-looking hands.

Daily maintenance
- Cuticles and nails will be soft directly after a bath or shower, so take advantage of this. Gently ease under cuticles and nail tips with a hoof stick to remove dead skin and debris. Trim away any loose skin flaps with nail scissors.
- When you apply body lotion, work it into your hands too. Gently train cuticles away from nails by stroking firmly back with the pad of your thumb.

Weekly maintenance
- The best time to file is also when nails are damp and less likely to split. Use a fine-textured emery board and use long, sweeping strokes from sides to centre – don't saw back and forth. Shape the tip to echo the curve of the nail base, but don't file too far down at the sides – this weakens stress points and causes splits. Seal the nail layers and prevent the tips from flaking by lightly flicking the extra-fine side of the emery forwards along the nail.
- Buff the nails with a smooth buffer. This boosts the circulation, helps even out ridges, seals nail tips and leaves a natural, healthy-looking sheen. Finish with a helping of handcream.
- Long nails look awful on older hands. Short nails are more flattering and less likely to break or split. The ideal length is just beyond the fingertips, so that the 'white' edges can be shaped to echo the curve of the half-moons at the base.

FEET

Take the strain off your hardest workers – check out your shoes! Chiropodists estimate that 75 per cent of foot problems are caused by constantly wearing high heels which force toes forwards, over-arch the feet and impose the entire body weight on the heels and balls of the feet. Burning sensations on the balls of the feet are caused by the foot sliding into the narrowest part of the shoe and are early warning signs of hard skin build-up. Corns and calluses ultimately form to protect the bones and joints from this type of shock.

- Alternate your footwear to relieve pressure and keep muscles and tendons flexible. A low heel of around 2.5–5cm (1–2 inches) is often more comfortable than totally flat, as the slightly raised heel is less likely to jar. Keep high heels for evenings only.
- When you're running, walking or exercising, always wear trainers with good, shock-absorbing soles.
- To exercise feet, chiropodists recommend walking barefoot around the house, or more pleasurably, on the beach. Gripping damp sand works the toes and acts as a natural dead skin exfoliator.
- Moisturize feet daily, especially in summer. Open sandals mean perspiration evaporates fast and skin easily gets tough and cracked, especially around the heels.

Moisturizing foot massage

Prevent hard skin build-up and keep feet comfortably smooth. Carry out this routine when feet are softened after a bath or shower.
- Rub off dead skin from around the heels and balls of the feet and under the big toe with a pumice stone. Don't use metal files – they can irritate and damage tender skin.
- Gently massage exfoliating cream or damp sea salt all over

the feet, using circular fingertip movements. Ease back cuticles and clean under the nail tip with an orange stick. Rinse and blot dry.

- Trim the nails with a toenail clipper. Cut straight across to prevent splitting and ingrowing nails. Buff edges smooth with the fine side of an emery board. Use the rough side to fine-tune hard skin around the toes. Rinse and dry thoroughly, especially between the toes.
- Massage a moisturizing cream over the feet, paying special care to the heels. Add a drop of antibacterial peppermint oil to your footcream to keep feet cool and fresh.

TEN-MINUTE TIP

Flex feet and trim ankles

You can do these exercises singly, but it's best to do them together whenever you can.

- Point the foot and rotate each ankle ten times in both directions. This helps to beat fluid retention and reduces puffiness.
- Flex the foot up and back. Hold for ten seconds, then relax. Repeat 15 times per foot.
- Shape and tone the calves. Put a thick book on the floor or stand on the bottom stair. Position the front half of your feet on the 'step' and gently raise and lower the heels. Repeat 30 times, using a chairback or the banister for balance.
- Practise picking up a pencil with your toes. It is difficult at first, but it does keep your toes supple and improves their grip and thus your balance and posture.

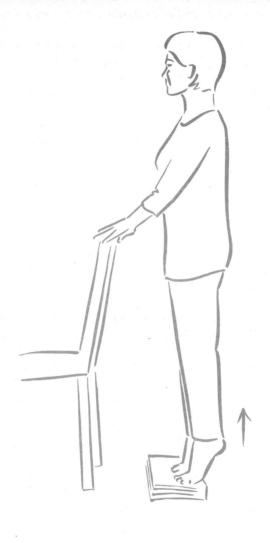

CHAPTER 8

Youth foods
Eating yourself younger

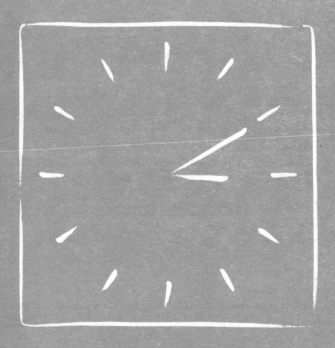

Dieting can be dangerous. There is growing evidence to suggest that an obsession with weight control may mean we're malnourished. If we deny ourselves the full range of nutrients our body needs to function well, we lessen our chances of staying fit, healthy and younger-looking. Here's how to eat your way to natural weight control and peak vitality.

Never say 'never too thin'. Certainly obesity is a health hazard. But for women, controlled curves are healthier than skinny limbs, especially from middle age onwards. According to a study at St Thomas's Hospital in London, pear-shaped women with generous bottoms and thighs are less likely to suffer heart disease and diabetes than their 'straight up and down' sisters. But beware of a bulging tummy – the type of fat that collects around the waistline constantly breaks down and circulates in the blood, posing increased risk of heart disease, high blood pressure and diabetes.

Strict dieting is not the successful and lasting answer to weight control. Our food intake is down 20 per cent on ten years ago, yet obesity rates have doubled. Why? In our labour-saving, couch-hugging culture of cars, lifts and mail order shopping, we're simply gaining weight faster than we burn calories. Skipping main meals and snacking on 'empty calorie' junk foods is yet another major factor in stealthy weight gain. Cutting down means reducing our food intake, but as we grow older, the body increases its need for essential nutrients to maintain the immune system. The right approach, then, is to boost our quota of quality food and balance it with exercise.

SUPERNUTRIENTS – THE FOODS THAT FIGHT AGEING

One of the most popular theories as to why and how we age is that of free radical damage. Free radicals are molecules with an unpaired or missing electron which they try to snatch from any other molecule. Free radicals are by-products of oxygen combustion – that's breathing – and our body needs a certain amount of them to fight infection. But 'superoxide' molecules can get out of control and attack cells, turning their lipids rancid, hard and unable to absorb nutrients until eventually, they die.

What combats free radicals? Chemical compounds and enzymes called antioxidants protect cells by 'pairing up' with free radicals instead. The body produces its own antioxidants which repair about 99 per cent of daily damage, but the remaining 1 per cent accrues with age. Cell damage hastens the ageing process, increasing the risk of age-related illness. It's estimated that by the age of 50, 30 per cent of our cellular protein has been damaged by free radical activity, and 80–90 per cent of diseases such as cancer, heart disease, arthritis and Alzheimer's are caused by free radical damage. Is there anything we can do to prevent free radical overload? Protect yourself from 'oxidizing' environments – cigarette smoke, pollution and sunlight all excite free radical activity. Avoid heavily processed and smoked foods and

The body produces its own antioxidants which repair about 99 per cent of daily damage

eat foods rich in antioxidants. As an extra precaution, take antioxidant supplements wisely.

WHY TAKE SUPPLEMENTS?

If you eat a balanced diet, you don't need to supplement it with pills, so the orthodox argument goes. Yet many nutritionists now argue that eating refined foods and fruit and vegetables that are less than fresh can mean we may not be sufficiently nourished to withstand increasing levels of free radical attack from the environment. Some cooking methods can destroy nutrients, too. Boiling leaches out some vitamins, while frying and char-grilling generate free radicals. Our age, sex, stress levels and lifestyle also determine how much nutrients we need and use. American health and nutrition expert Jean Carper argues that although a varied and wisely balanced diet is the launching pad to good health, it's no longer smart to think food can give you all the vitamins and minerals you need to combat early ageing. We may think we're meeting the RDAs – Recommended Dietary Allowances for vitamins and minerals set by each country's government – but RDA levels reflect only the amounts necessary to prevent deficiency diseases and are, say many experts, badly out of date. In terms of peak health they're hopelessly low, says Jean Carper, and she's not alone.

Dr Denham Harman, Emeritus Professor of Medicine at the University of Nebraska College of Medicine, was the first to propose the free radical theory of ageing in back in 1954. He takes this anti-ageing cocktail daily: vitamin E – 150–300 international units (IU); vitamin C – 2000mg taken in four 500mg doses; coenzyme Q10 – 30mg, taken in 10mg doses three times a day; selenium – 100 micrograms taken in 50mcg doses twice daily; magnesium – 250mg; and a low-dose multivitamin and mineral tablet without iron. Every other day, he also takes

25,000IU (15mg) beta-carotene and 30mg zinc. Sounds like a lot to swallow? Earl Stadtman, PhD, Chief of the Laboratory of Biochemistry at the National Heart, Lung and Blood Institute in the USA, takes a daily antioxidant trio of 400IU vitamin E, 500mg vitamin C and 25,000IU beta carotene.

But good nutrition relies on balance, so for most of us who aren't quite sure what we're doing, prebalanced antioxidant formulas are the safest best. Look for ones that include vitamins A, beta-carotene, C and E, plus minerals such as zinc, copper, manganese and selenium – and stick to the recommended daily dose. A single daily multivitamin and mineral pill can also substantially boost your nutrient quota and is a balanced starting point for safe supplementation.

ANTIOXIDANT ALLIES

VITAMIN A AND BETA-CAROTENE (PRO-VITAMIN A)

Vitamin A, or retinol, is vital for strong skin, teeth, bones and mucous membranes. The body converts beta-carotene from food into vitamin A as and when needed. Studies show that beta-carotene can lower the risk of heart disease and cancers including breast and cervical. It may also help to protect against ultraviolet light, shielding us to some extent from wrinkles and skin cancer, and against cataracts.

Beta-carotene can lower the risk of heart disease and cancers

Dose: the EC RDA for retinol is 800mcg (UK RDA is 600mcg for women; 700mcg for men). It is toxic above 25,000IU. The Department of Health has recommended that women who are, or may be, pregnant should not take dietary supplements containing vitamin A except on the advice of their doctor. There is no RDA for beta-carotene, but six units gives one of retinol – a 3mg dose equals 5000IU of vitamin A. Its upper safe level is 20mg.

Food sources: retinol is found in fish, meat, dairy products and eggs. Beta-carotene comes from dark green or orange foods like broccoli, spinach, carrots, apricots, peaches and sweet potato.

VITAMIN C

This is a potent antioxidant that many studies suggest can help prevent cancer. It raises levels of glutathione in the blood, meaning it also protects cells from free radical damage and premature ageing. It may also prevent viral infection and cataracts and lessen the effects of pollution, smoking and allergic reactions. It is vital for the formation of collagen protein, which keeps skin firm and plump.

Dose: the EC RDA is 60mg (UK RDA is 40mg) and 100mg for smokers, but most experts recommend a daily maintenance dose of at least 1000mg (1g) and 6000mg to fight infections like colds and flu. High doses cause diarrhoea, though. Calcium ascorbate crystals are gentler on the stomach and easier to tolerate than regular ascorbic acid.

Food sources: guava, mango, kiwi fruit, grapefruit, broccoli, cantaloupe, strawberry, red pepper, sweet potato, sugar snap peas, oranges, cherries, blackcurrants.

VITAMIN E

Currently one of the 'hottest' antioxidants, it has been called the body's first line of defence against lipid peroxidation. It protects fatty acids in cells from free radical attack and works in synergy with selenium, another important anti-ageing antioxidant. Studies have linked vitamin E with the prevention of heart disease as it can lower LDL cholesterol and prevent its oxidation, thin the blood and prevent clots. There is growing evidence that it may protect against various cancers, including lung cancer. In cases of maturity-onset diabetes which occurs at mid-life and beyond, some studies show that vitamin E may help to improve insulin use and help regulate blood sugar levels. It may reduce anxiety and depression, enhance skin condition and the immune response, and prevent cataracts. There is also anecdotal evidence that it may slow greying hair.

Dose: the EC RDA is 10mg or 14.9IU (there is no UK RDA for vitamin E). Studies show 100–200IU reduces the risk of heart disease and some experts recommend up to 400IU. But avoid supplements if you take a blood thinner such as aspirin or warfarin. Supplements should also be avoided in iron deficiency anaemia.

Food sources: vegetable oils, sweet potato, wheatgerm, nuts, avocado pears and sunflower seeds.

BIOFLAVONOIDS

These give colour to fruit and vegetables and work with vitamin C to keep connective tissue healthy and improve capillary strength. Rutin can prevent bleeding gums and varicose veins; quercetin protects against heart disease and cancer. Bioflavonoids are believed to have antiviral activity, especially in combination with vitamin C.

Dose: no RDA. The usual combination with vitamin C is 500mg vitamin C to 100mg bioflavonoids. Take 1000mg bioflavonoids to 400–800IUs of vitamin D.

Food sources: pith and segments of citrus fruits, apricots, buckwheat, red and yellow onions, blackberries, cherries, rose hips, tea and apples.

SELENIUM

This mineral works with vitamin E to curb inflammatory diseases such as arthritis. Population studies show that cancer death rates are directly linked to the amount of selenium absorbed from the diet. There is also evidence suggesting selenium helps protect against heart disease by preventing lipids from clogging arteries and blood clots which cause strokes and heart attacks. Studies have also shown selenium boosts the immune system.

Dose: no EC RDA (UK RDA is 75µg for men and 60µg for women). 'Anti-ageing' health experts recommend 100µg daily. The Department of Health have set an upper limit of 450µg per day, but the dose from supplements should not exceed 200µg per day.

Food sources: Selenium levels in soils vary according to region, affecting its richness in foods such as wheatgerm, brazil nuts, pine nuts, sesame seeds, sunflower seeds and poppy seeds. Fish and liver are also good sources.

THE BEST ANTI-AGEING FOODS

These antioxidant fruits and vegetables are foods we should feast on daily to fight ageing. Enjoy them raw for their full protective potency.

- **Avocado** is rich in vitamin E. It also contains potassium which helps control blood pressure.

- **Berries.** Strawberries, raspberries, cranberries and blueberries are rich in vitamin C. Blueberries are the richest source of antioxidant anthocyanins.
- **Broccoli** is rich in antioxidants vitamin C, beta-carotene, quercetin, indoles, glutathione and lutein. It helps to guard against lung cancer, colon and cardiovascular disease and may have a role in preventing breast cancer by neutralizing excess oestrogen.
- **Cabbage** contains indole-3-carbinol, which helps to prevent breast cancer and lowers the risk of colonic and stomach cancers.
- **Carrots** help to lower cholesterol and reduce the risk of stroke and lung and stomach cancer. They may also be beneficial for age-related eye disease and failing eyesight.
- **Citrus fruits.** Oranges contain powerful cancer-fighting carotenoids, terpenes, flavonoids and vitamin C and may help reduce the risk of cataracts and cancer.
- **Grapes** contain at least 20 known antioxidants. Richly coloured types are the most potent; raisins are more powerful than fresh grapes. Grape antioxidants strengthen blood vessels and prevent cholesterol build up and heart disease. Oligomeric proanthocyanadin complexes (OPCs) in grapeseeds are said to prevent collagen cross-linking which causes slack skin.
- **Garlic** contains at least a dozen antioxidants plus ajoene which helps prevent blood clots; and allicin, a natural antiviral, antifungal and antibacterial agent which helps reduce cholesterol levels, and may prevent artery and heart disease. Garlic also stimulates immune function.
- **Onions**, like garlic, help to prevent blood clots by raising 'good' HDL cholesterol levels. Red and yellow types are richest in cancer-inhibiting quercetin, which also has anti-inflammatory, antibacterial, antifungal and antiviral properties.
- **Spinach** contains beta-carotene and lutein, both powerful

antioxidants which help protect against cancer, heart disease, high blood pressure, strokes, cataracts and macular degeneration which can cause blindness. It also contains folic acid, which helps protect against birth defects such as spina bifida, and also heart disease.

- **Tea**, and especially green tea, is now billed the 'longevity' drink which helps prevent heart disease and cancer, thanks to antioxidants such as polyphenols, quercetin and catechins.
- **Tomatoes** are the richest and most reliable source of lycopene, an extremely potent antioxidant that helps protect against prostate and possibly breast cancer. It also helps preserve physical and mental functions, especially in the elderly. Research suggests tomatoes may also guard against heart disease, especially when cooked.

SMART SUPPLEMENTS – WHICH SHOULD YOU BE TAKING?

Not a month goes by these days without some 'wonder pill' hitting the headlines. No single nutrient has been proved to stop the clock, but some may help offset specific age-related problems. Remember to take your choice as part of a balanced diet and with a good multivitamin and mineral formula. If you are taking medication for a particular health problem, talk to your GP about your plan to take supplements. These are six of the best.

COENZYME Q10 (UBIQUINONE)

This converts energy from food into a form that the body can store and use for both physical and mental activity. It is found in oily fish, wholegrain cereals, nuts, meat and vegetables. CoQ10 is believed to strengthen heart muscle, protect against heart disease and cancer, and can be beneficial in treating gingivitis. Swedish research compares CoQ10's antioxidant powers to vitamin E, which protects cells against damage and degenerative disease. Experiments with mice at the New England Institute showed CoQ10 not only increased their lifespan by 50 per cent, they remained bright-eyed, glossy-coated and sprightly.

DHEA (DEHYDROEPIANDROSTERONE)

DHEA is a hormone-like substance which is produced largely by the adrenal glands but also in smaller quantities by the ovaries. It is converted into oestrogen, progesterone, testos-terone and cortisone. With age, DHEA levels decline and by the age of 60 it's barely detectable in women. Animal studies indicate that high-level supplements boost energy, memory and libido and may protect against heart disease, osteopor osis, cancer, depression and aggression. Alzheimer's and breast cancer sufferers have been found to be deficient in DHEA, suggesting it may be useful in protecting against those diseases too. However, most experts point out that not enough is known yet about DHEA for over-the-counter sales. Side-effects of large doses are an enlarged liver and facial hair in women. It's also known that some forms of breast cancer are linked with excess hormones in the body. Nevertheless, some doctors prescribe DHEA as part of the HRT mix, finding they need to use less oestrogen because the body converts DHEA into both oestrogen and libido-restoring testosterone. Wild yam (see below) is a natural source of DHEA.

DONG QUAI

What we know as angelica is the premier Chinese remedy for PMS and is also called the 'female ginseng'. A natural adapto-gen, it balances the menstrual cycle, preventing cramps, bloating, acne and irritability. Its weak levels of plant oestrogens can dilute excess oestrogen in the body, or augment it when levels are low. It helps to regulate the cycle after coming off the Pill, and reduces hot flushes, vaginal dryness and palpitations during menopause. It is also rich in iron and the antioxidant vitamin E. According to some studies, dong quai can lower blood pressure, regulate blood sugar and help prevent anaemia.

GINKGO BILOBA

In China, this tree is called the plant of youth. The heart-shaped leaves and plum-like seeds are used to treat respiratory ailments, such as tuberculosis, asthma, bronchitis and circulatory problems. In the West, its ability to boost blood and oxygen flow to the extremities and brain has caught the imagination of scientists. Studies indicate that ginkgo's powerful antioxidants dilate blood vessels, may help to prevent strokes and speed brain tissue repair. In 1994, the *Lancet* officially backed ginkgo's use in treating circulatory diseases, including Raynaud's disease. Studies have also shown it helps to combat memory loss and boost concentration.

> *In 1994, the Lancet officially backed ginko's use in treating circulatory diseases, including Raynaud's disease*

GINSENG

The Chinese have used this famous root for 5000 years as a rejuvenating cure-all. It is said to improve memory and mental performance, especially in older people. Japanese studies have found that it contains antioxidants that inhibit the growth of cancer cells and lower cholesterol, while Russian studies have demonstrated its ability to fight stress by normalizing body functions such as blood sugar and pressure levels. It is also believed to improve libido and sexual vigour, and to have aphrodisiac properties.

GLUTATHIONE

Glutathione is a powerful antioxidant which is synthesized in the body from three other amino acids – L-cysteine, L-glutamic acid and glycine, all found in fruits and vegetables such as citrus fruits, melon and raw carrots. Studies have shown that it may help protect against cancer, radiation and debilitation due to smoking and alcohol abuse. It is a popular supplement in Japan, where the average lifespan is the longest in the world. It has major detoxifying properties and a recent study at the Human Nutrition Research Center on Ageing at Tufts University in the USA suggests that supplements may help to keep an ageing immune system healthy. Other studies indicate that glutathione may act as an anti-inflammatory agent and may prove useful in reducing the symptoms of allergies and arthritis.

MELATONIN

This hormone is secreted by the pineal gland in the brain during sleep. It is crucial to body rhythms, especially the circadian rhythm, which regulates sleep–wake cycles. Widely used to ease the symptoms of jet lag, it can also help cure insomnia. Production of melatonin drops dramatically with age. At 65, we have a quarter of the natural melatonin we had at 25 – one reason at least why a growing number of researchers suspect it may be a key anti-ageing hormone. Animal studies have shown that removing the pineal gland accelerates the ageing process, while melatonin supplementation can prolong life by 20 per cent. Some researchers believe melatonin is a natural anti-ager due to powerful antioxidant properties; others say it can 'time release' other hormones, proteins and neurotransmitters vital for cell communication. It is available over the counter in the US, but not in the UK.

WILD YAM

This increasingly popular 'anti-ageing' vegetable extract is a traditional African folk remedy for rheumatoid arthritis and colic. Herbalists also prescribe it to ease PMS and menopausal symptoms such as hot flushes, fatigue and vaginal dryness – hence its reputation as the alternative HRT. Scientists first extracted the hormone progesterone from wild yam in 1943, and until 1970 it was the sole source of this hormone for the contraceptive pill.

What is a balanced diet?

Good food is the closest thing to a 'youth drug'. Follow the British Government's National Food Guide and eat the right amounts from each of the following food groups each day. This will ensure you get the full range of essential vitamins and minerals your body needs to maintain good health.

- Bread, potatoes and cereals: 34 per cent.
- Vegetables and fruit: 33 per cent.
- Dairy products: 15 per cent.
- Meat, fish and alternative proteins: 12 per cent.
- Fatty and sugary foods: 6 per cent.

Timing meals right

Eat throughout the day to maintain blood sugar levels for energy and alertness. Spacing meals well may also help reduce the temptation to snack – and if you consume calories consistently your body uses them more efficiently so there's less risk of gaining weight.

- *Morning*. Eat a substantial breakfast first thing. Snack on fruit mid-morning.
- *Midday*. Try to have lunch around 12 o'clock and not later than 1 p.m. Then, mid-afternoon, nibble nuts or a slice of wholemeal bread.
- *Evening*. Keep dinner light and preferably before 8 p.m.

> *If you consume calories consistently your body uses them more efficiently*

BONING UP

Thinning bones is one of the biggest health threats to women after the menopause. One in three women (and one in twelve men) is likely to develop osteoporosis. Signs are a rounded back and a 'dowager's hump' at the back of the neck. More seriously, osteoporosis makes bones – especially spinal, hip and wrist – vulnerable to fractures and breaks. By the age of 30, peak bone mass has developed and the production of new bone cells starts to slow. After 35, bones begin to lose around 1 per cent bone mass annually, rising to 2–4 per cent yearly after the menopause.

Declining levels of oestrogen, which in women is essential for the absorption of the bone mineral calcium, cause osteoporosis. Hormone replacement therapy (HRT) halts rapid bone loss, but may not be suitable for all women – and once HRT is stopped, bone loss accelerates again. Good nutrition before, during and after the menopause is the natural solution. Soya bean products such as tofu and soya milk contain genistein, a rich source of plant oestrogens which mimic the body's natural hormones. Weight-bearing exercise, including walking and jogging, builds bones and boosts muscle mass which could help cushion a fall, and it has been shown that combining exercise with vitamin and mineral supplementation can significantly lower the risk of osteoporosis. These are your key bone boosters.

VITAMIN D

This is essential to allow the body to use calcium and phosphorus. Sunlight stimulates certain skin oils to synthesize vitamin D in the body, but consistently using high factor sunblocks could inhibit this natural process. Expose some area of your skin – eg hands or arms – to daylight for ten minutes twice a day; double for black and Asian skins.

Foods: dairy products and oily fish. Fortified margarines.
Supplements: the EC RDA for vitamin D is 5μg. There is some evidence that 400IUs during winter, when bone loss is most rapid, can reduce the loss. Toxicity level is over 50μg daily.

CALCIUM

This mineral allows bones to reach their peak mass and maintain their strength and density. It's thought that maintaining good calcium levels throughout the thirties, forties and fifties builds reserves to draw upon later.

Foods: low-fat dairy products – an average (150g) tub of plain yoghurt contains around 285mg of calcium. However, some low-fat cheeses contain phosphate, which inhibits calcium absorption. Tofu processed with calcium sulphate, sardines with bones, and broccoli are all good sources.
Supplements: the EC RDA for calcium is 800mg (UK RDA is 700mg). Some experts recommend up to the upper safe level of 1500mg for post-menopausal women not on HRT. Calcium carbonate delivers most efficiently.

BORON

Research suggests that boron can reduce the loss of calcium and magnesium, both needed to build and maintain strong bones.

Foods: many fruits, vegetables and nuts, especially dried prunes and apricots.
Supplements: take 3mg daily (do not take more than 10mg). It works best combined with a good vitamin and mineral supplement including calcium, magnesium, manganese and riboflavin.

Drinking to long life

- **Alcohol.** Wine, especially red wine, contains antioxidants which reduce LDL cholesterol and therefore reduce the risk of heart disease. Women past the menopause who drink small amounts of wine daily are less likely to develop heart problems. Up to two units or measures daily gives the maximum benefit and won't risk your health. But watch it – an average glass of wine packs around 95 calories.
- **Water.** It's calorie-free and a better thirst-quencher than soft fizzy drinks which are riddled with sugars and additives. Professor Don Naismith, Emeritus Professor of Nutrition at King's College, recommends drinking 1.8 litres ($3^1/_4$ pints) daily to prevent dehydration. Other experts recommend up to 3 litres ($5^1/_4$ pints) in hot weather or while playing sports. However, there is little evidence that drinking more benefits skin, and some dermatologists believe that skin becomes puffy and spongy from H_2O abuse.
- **Fruit and vegetable juices.** These are also preferable to soft drinks. They supply antioxidant vitamins and minerals. It's best to squeeze them fresh yourself, but if you buy them avoid sweetened commercial brands.
- **Tea and coffee.** Whilst they contain stimulants that pick you up initially, they wear you down eventually if you drink them all day. Limit coffee to one cup maximum, preferably in the morning. Tea offers antioxidants, but too much tannin may inhibit iron absorption. Herb teas are refreshing and have other therapeutic properties such as calming the nerves or aiding respiration and digestion.

FAT FACTS

In our quest to stay fit, slim and younger-looking we've become fat phobics. But cutting out fat also risks health. If a woman's fat intake falls below 15 per cent of her total calorie intake daily, her oestrogen levels fall, leading to menstrual problems, osteoporosis and fatigue. There are also some fats that are essential – hence their name, Essential Fatty Acids (EFAs). As well as maintaining hormonal balance, EFAs are needed for healthy blood vessels, nerves and skin cells. They help prevent heart disease by controlling cholesterol and boost calcium absorption – yet another way of ensuring healthy bones. EFAs also help combat dry skin and keep hair glossy. Make sure you get a good balance of these EFAs in your diet.

Omega-3 is vital for good brain function and eyesight and prevents inflammation and blood clotting. It also helps to prevent heart and bowel disease and breast cancer. Get it from sunflower, safflower and linseed oils, nuts and oily fish such as mackerel, salmon, herring and cod.

Omega-6 works with Omega-3 to regulate the production of prostaglandins – hormone-like substances that control inflammation and blood pressure. You can obtain it from seeds, vegetables, sunflower, safflower and sesame oils. Evening primrose oil is a rich source which helps with PMS and menopausal problems, sore breasts and skin inflammation. But be careful – too much Omega-6 is also linked with arthritis, strokes, diabetes and some types of cancer.

FAT MANAGEMENT

Here's the healthy way to include fats in your diet.

- The World Health Organization recommends that 20 per cent fat or 40g per 2000 calories is healthy for women, so long as no more than 10 per cent of that is saturated fat.
- EFAs should provide at least one-third of the total fat in your diet.

- Avoid saturated animal fats, hydrogenated fats in processed foods, and margarines containing trans-fats, which increase the risk of heart disease by boosting levels of artery-clogging LDL cholesterol. Animal fats have also been linked to breast and colon cancer and rheumatoid arthritis. A dangerous source of free radicals, they may also hasten premature ageing.

TEN-MINUTE TIP

Cheers!

Beta-Brews: raw fruit and vegetable juices supply undiluted nutrient 'shots' to the system. Choose fresh, preferably organic produce and drink the juice the minute it's processed. Enjoy these antioxidant recipes daily for a firm, glowing skin which resists premature wrinkles. In a juicer, put:

$1^1/_2$ large carrots, scrubbed
125g (4oz) spinach
1 apple with peel

or

4 apricots
150g (5oz) strawberries
1 orange, peel, pith removed

For extra benefits, add a tablespoon of wheatgerm for vitamins E and B group and mashed avocado or banana, both rich sources of minerals, especially potassium.

CHAPTER 9

Exercise
Becoming your own powerhouse

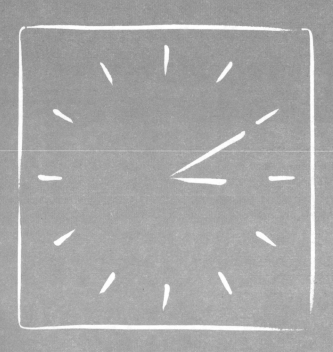

Your body is a machine that's designed to keep moving; stop for long periods and it simply loses its power to stay fully mobile. A sedentary lifestyle is linked to a variety of diseases, especially in later years, and experts estimate that keeping fit can extend life by approximately two years. Most mobility problems in old age have middle-age origins – being unfit at 40 stores up problems for later. But the best news is that it's never too late to get off the couch. And remember, any form of movement, from dancing to yoga, counts as healthy exercise, as long as you keep it up. Choose a move you enjoy – and go for it!

GYM MOVES

Gym classes encourage commitment – a major plus in their favour. If you've never joined a gym in your life before, you may be in for a pleasant surprise. The current fitness boom means you're unlikely to feel the odd slob out – all body shapes and sizes will be there, not only the slim and dauntingly superfit. Qualified instructors will also ensure you work out effectively and safely for your personal fitness level, which should be assessed before you start any training programme. Experts recommend 'cross-training' — combining different kinds of classes for all-round stamina, strength, fat-busting and firming. For example, aerobic training burns calories, while strength work boosts muscle mass. Combining yoga stretches with aerobic exercise is becoming increasingly popular with those who wish to maximize balance and flexibility. These are the most popular classes.

AEROBICS

These offer cardiovascular fitness, calorie-burning and co-ordination. Routine, high-energy exercises are designed to get your heart pumping. Least stressful on the back and knee joints are low-impact aerobics, where one foot always remains on the ground. Most classes also include stretching and spot toning moves.

BODY CONDITIONING

Take body conditioning classes for strength, tone and suppleness. Warm-ups often include low-impact aerobics. The main moves are a specific sequence of toning exercises involving hand weights, rubber tubing or the resistance of your own body weight.

CIRCUIT TRAINING

This is for all-round fitness, strength and flexibility. You move around the gym doing various exercises, such as press-ups, sit-ups, squats and benchwork. Aerobic exercises are often included in classes, as is the use of equipment such as skipping ropes and hand weights. Circuit training with Nautilus equipment and exercise machines — bikes, treadmills, stair machines and the various machines that use weight resistance to tone specific body muscles – gives fast results. By the end of the session, all body zones will have been worked.

WALKING – THE NATURAL WORKOUT

Walking is the most basic form of aerobic exercise and potentially the most rewarding. After the tyrannical 'going for the burn' philosophy that dominated the 1980s, current exercise trends favour more achievable and sustainable activities. Formerly frenzied joggers have slowed down to low-impact but high-energy power-walking to and from work. It's because walking can be so easily included in everyone's lifestyle that makes it so appealing.

Power or brisk walking burns around 100 calories per mile, while freeing up stiff joints and boosting cardiovascular performance. Wherever you walk, wear comfortable supportive trainers and, ideally, layers of loose clothing you can peel off and put back on as your body temperature changes.

Walking can also train you into better posture. In the USA, movement teacher Suki Munsell has developed her own posture-perfect Dynamic Walking programme.

• First, check in the mirror how you stand. Imagine a line running from each ear through your shoulder, hip and knee down to your ankle. Relax your shoulder and elongate your lower back. Don't lock your knees – just be aware of your pelvis comfortably supporting your upper body.
• Now start to walk, noticing any aches, pains and stiffness. Analyse your stride. Make sure your feet are parallel and don't roll either to the inside or the outside and that your steps – from heel-strike through foot-flex to push-off – are similar on both feet. Make sure your hips move evenly on both sides too.
• For perfect posture, lift your spine out of your hips and let

your lower back relax and lengthen. Imagine you have a heavy tail and that the top of your head is stretching to receive a crown.

WATER WORKOUTS

Swimming is nearly the perfect all-round toner. A highly aerobic exercise, it works all body zones evenly and hard, and the body burns extra calories to keep warm in cold water. Swimming is ideal physiotherapy that tones muscles without straining or jolting joints, as the water provides resistance – it is around 1000 times denser than air – but eradicates impact. Your body is 90 per cent lighter in the water, which is one good reason why beginners, the elderly, the overweight and pregnant women have made aqua-aerobics an increasingly popular alternative to land-locked classes. Try jogging or walking across the width of the pool, keeping your pelvis tilted forwards and your stomach muscles pulled in, to see how hard water can make you work.

When you swim, kicking stretches the thigh and buttock muscles, simultaneously elongating and toning them, and the breast stroke kick is especially good for the inner thighs. But although swimming is a no-impact, weightless workout, continual laps of breaststroke can strain the knee joints, neck and back. Alexander Technique teachers warn against holding the head up out of the water while swimming breaststroke – it's the postural equivalent of walking with your face turned to the sky, they say, and done frequently it can compromise spinal alignment. To swim safely and well, you have to be prepared to get your face and hair wet. Wear goggles to protect your eyes from chlorine. Raise your head only to breathe in, then blow out hard into the water to prevent it from getting up your nose or into your mouth. Vary your stroke. Backstroke and crawl relieve the tension of breaststroke and work the arms harder. Ideally, repeat the three strokes in the lap sequences.

Aquarobics – or water exercise – works bits of you the gym can often miss. Water provides resistance but takes the strain off shockable joints, so muscles are toned without risk of strain – an invaluable plus-point for those who suffer stiffness or arthritis. Aquafit exercises improve co-ordination, stamina, muscle and cardiovascular tone. For the overweight or inactive, gentle water exercise helps to rebuild and maintain tone and fitness, while helping to control oedema – puffiness and swelling in the ankles and feet. Asthma sufferers benefit too, as swimming helps to control the frequency of your breathing.

To boost your general heart rate and fitness level, try these exercises. Remember, speed increases water-resistance – the faster you try to go, the more intense your workout. For even greater water resistance, change direction frequently.

- **Water walking.** Walk the lap to boost heart rate and work buttocks and backs and front of thighs. Keep the back straight and relaxed and the stomach muscles tucked in, then try jogging.
- **On-the-spot jogging.** Jog, raising your knees as high as you can. Keep your balance and work your arms at the same time. Turn your palms to the front and pull them up to water level. Now push your palms down and back against the water.
- **Star-jumps.** To tone inner and outer thighs, stand with your feet hip-width apart, tummy tucked in. Jump apart, bounce, then jump feet together and bounce. Your arms should mirror your legs below the water surface to work upper and lower muscles.
- **Stomach crunchers.** Grip the side of the pool with both hands, shoulder-width apart. Draw your knees slowly up to your chest then shoot them down and slightly backwards to toe-touch the bottom. Repeat as fast as you can, breathing in as you raise your knees and out as you straighten your

legs. You should feel your stomach muscles tightening.

- **Water-skis.** This exercise trims the waist. With your feet together, start facing front, then bounce from the hips to either side, keeping your upper body straight. Swing your arms in the opposite direction to your feet for balance.

WHY EXERCISE?

- **For mobility.** Keeping active means maintaining your full range of movements. Joints seize up with disuse. Blood is pumped to the joints when they're in use; if they're not, cartilage deteriorates and joints stiffen.
- **For stamina.** Cardiovascular activity gets lazy during periods of inertia. Inactive muscles demand less blood and oxygen than the heart and lungs are capable of supplying.
- **For strength.** Sedentary muscles waste quickly and tire sooner. Strength generates strength.
- **For general health.** Exercise can prevent heart disease. Blood composition changes with inactivity; clogging LDL cholesterol levels rise and scouring HDL cholesterol drops. As clotting factors increase, the blood gets thicker and stickier. Exercise lowers blood pressure, boosts circulation and also helps to prevent diabetes. Weight-bearing exercise generates bone mass and so prevents osteoporosis; American studies have found evidence of bone thinning in inactive women as young as their early forties. An activity as simple as carrying evenly weighted shopping bags in both hands can strengthen wrists. Weight machines in the gym are designed to provide resistance while limiting the strain factor.
- **For relaxation.** Exercise not only liberates tense muscles, it lightens the mind by working off nervous tension. You don't have to go for the burn for endorphins, the body's natural opiates, to be released into the bloodstream for a

pleasantly natural high. Exercise can be a potent antidote to depression – you feel a real sense of achievement which raises your self-esteem. Regular exercise generates more energy during the day and better quality sleep at night and is a natural remedy for insomnia. Aerobic exercise also contributes to mental alertness, thanks to the increased supply of oxygen to the brain.

- **For weight control.** With age, body fat increases and muscle ratio diminishes. The reason for this is most likely to be increasing inactivity. With exercise, fat stores decline, muscle tone builds, metabolic rate increases and your shape is improved. Exercise is a far more healthy and successful way of progressively losing weight than dieting – although starting a fitness routine often brings the incentive to streamline your diet, too.

YOUR TOP TEN AGE-ZONE TONERS

The workout that hits the troublespots

These ten daily toners all tackle zones most hit by age. Pick the ones you need most to build into your own ten-minute daily workout programme.

WARM-UP AND WIND-DOWN

Prevent strain and muscle injury with gentle stretching and flexing moves before and after exercise. Hold each stretch for 15–20 seconds.

- **Loosen neck and shoulders.** Stand straight with your feet shoulder-width apart. Relax your shoulders back and down. Very gently tilt your head to the right, feeling your neck stretch. Hold for 10 seconds, then tilt to the left and hold. Centre your head. Raise your right shoulder up towards your ear. Rotate back, down and up again three full times, then repeat forwards. Repeat with the left shoulder.

- **Stretch arms.** Rest your right hand on the back of your neck. With your left hand, gently pull your right elbow back and down until you feel the stretch in your upper arm. Change arms and repeat.

- **Stretch shoulder muscles.** Clasp your hands loosely in front of you and raise arms straight out in front to shoulder level.

- **Stretch hamstrings.** Step forward with your left leg and straighten it. Keep your heel on the ground and raise your toes. Bend your right leg, keeping your heel on the floor. Keeping your back straight and relaxed, rest both hands on your right thigh and, keeping your weight on your back leg, ease into the stretch. Hold for 10 seconds. Change legs and repeat.

- **Stretch calves.** Step forward with your right leg, keeping your left leg straight. Both heels should be on the floor and toes pointing forward. Keep your back straight and hips to the front. Keeping your weight on your right leg, rest your hands on your right thigh, bend your knee and ease into the stretch. Hold for 10 seconds. Change legs and repeat.

- **Stretch thighs.** Stand on your right leg, gripping a chair with your right hand for balance if you need to. Keep your hips square, bend your left leg and catch the toes of your left foot with your free hand, easing it up towards your behind. Hold for 10 seconds. Change legs and repeat.

THE WORKOUT

1 *Trim a spare tyre.*
Stand with your feet shoulder-width apart, knees slightly bent. Rest your hands on your hips and keep your back straight and

shoulders down. Facing forwards, bend your torso to the right until you feel the stretch in your left side. Straighten up and repeat to the left. Repeat 15 times, building to 25 times each side.

2 *Flatten a flabby tum.*
Lie on your back, knees bent, feet flat on the floor hip-width apart. Supporting – but not pulling – your head with your hands, curl your upper body forwards off the ground. At the same time, breathe out and pull in with your stomach muscles. Slowly lower back to the start, breathing in. Repeat 10 times, building to 20 times.

3 *Tum toner two.*
Lie on your back, arms at your sides. Bend your knees and raise your legs up in the air, crossing your ankles. Breathe out and pull your stomach muscles in as you roll your hips up towards your ribs in a tiny, controlled movement. Hold for a count of 10 and breathe in. Then breathe out as you roll your hips back down. Always keep your back pressed to the floor. Repeat 10 times, building to 20 times.

4 *Tighten your bum.*
Kneel on all fours, keeping your knees below your hips and your elbows below your shoulders with your forearms forward

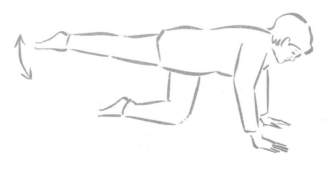

for balance. Straighten your right leg out behind you and lift it to hip level. Slowly lower. Keep your stomach muscles pulled in throughout this exercise. Repeat with the left leg. Repeat 15 times building to 25 times each leg.

5 *Lift 'sliding' bum, hips and thighs.*
Stand with your feet hip-width apart and stride forward with your right leg. Keeping your back straight and hips forward, slowly bend both knees until the left almost touches the floor behind you and the right leg is at right angles. Feel the stretch, then slowly straighten. Repeat, reversing your legs. Repeat 10–15 times each leg.

6 *Smooth lumpy fronts of thighs.*
Holding a chair for support, stand straight and turn your legs out slightly from the hips so that your knees face outwards. Raise the right leg as high as you can in front of you, aiming for waist level. Lower slowly. Repeat with the left leg. Repeat 15–20 times each leg.

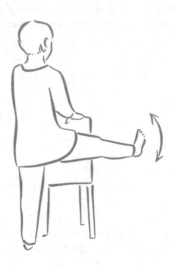

7 Firm saggy inner thighs.

Lie on your back, legs bent. Raise your knees to directly above your hips and lift your lower legs so that they are parallel to the ground. Press your back into the floor. Part your legs as far as you can to the sides then squeeze them back together. Rest your arms out at your sides for balance, or place your hands on your inner thighs for resistance. Repeat 15–20 times.

8 Tone saggy backs of arms.

Sit on a stool, back straight, stomach in, knees hip-width apart and feet flat on the floor. Hold a weight (450g/1lb building to 1.4kg/3lb) in your right hand, and raise towards the ceiling, straightening your arm. Place your left hand below your right elbow and, keeping your arm steady, lower the weight behind you until your elbow points upwards. Raise the weight to the ceiling again. Repeat, lowering the weight behind you 8 times. Swap arms. Repeat each set of 8 repetitions 3 times.

9 Firm front of arms and shrink 'bra overhang' at sides and back.

Sit on a stool and place a weight (450g/1lb building to 2.3kg/5lb) on the floor next to your right foot. Rest your left forearm over your thighs for support. Lean forwards, flattening your back. Pick up the weight with your right hand and draw it up to your armpit. Lead with your elbow and keep your arm close to your side. Slowly lower without letting the weight touch the floor. Repeat 8 times. Swap arms. Repeat each set of 8 repetitions 3 times.

10 Shape up sloping shoulders.

Stand with your feet hip-width apart, toes forward. Holding a weight (450g/1lb building to 1.4kg/3lb) in each hand, start with your hands in front of your thighs, palms inwards. Leading with your knuckles and keeping palms facing down, raise your arms out at the sides to shoulder level. Hold for a count of 5, then lower slowly. Repeat 8 times. Swap arms. Repeat each set of 8 repetitions 3 times.

Safe moves

- Exercise in a comfortably warm, well-ventilated room.
- Wear loose or flexible, comfortable clothes and trainers.
- Use a mat for floor exercises to protect your back, knees and elbows.
- Never exercise on a full stomach – wait for two hours after eating.
- Be motivated, but don't overdo it. Build up your repeats gradually and never force yourself into a position. If any exercise hurts, stop.
- Check with your doctor before beginning any exercise programme.

Success strategies

- Stay motivated – choose an exercise or sport you enjoy.
- Do it to music – it cuts the boredom factor and keeps you going longer. Choose a beat that paces you comfortably and realistically.
- Stay rhythmic – don't jerk or pull yourself into position. Movements should be fluid and controlled. Focusing on the muscles you are using helps.
- Breathe correctly – inhale with an active move like pulling in muscles or raising limbs. Exhale as you relax into a passive move.

SMART MOVES

Regular exercise builds and maintains all-round fitness and helps keep your weight stable. The calories burned in an hour of activity increase in proportion to your weight and how energetic your exercising is. Take this as a guide.

Action	Duration/ frequency	Calories burned per hour	Body benefits
IN THE GYM			
Aerobics	30–45 mins 2–3 times a week	Low impact: 200–300 High impact: 500–800	A total body tonic that improves the cardiovascular system.
Step class	30–45 mins 3 times a week	500–800	Tones and shapes legs; boosts strength and stamina and improves cardiovascular system.
Stretch	30–45 mins 2–3 times weekly	150	Improves flexibility gently.
Circuit training with weights	20–30 mins twice weekly	350–550	Tones and conditions muscles, boosts aerobic capacity.
SPORTS			
Tennis	30–40 mins 2–3 times weekly	400–1000	Strengthens lower body and shoulders. Improves cardiovascular system.
Squash	20–30 mins 2–3 times weekly	400–1000	As above.

Badminton	20–40 mins 2–3 times weekly	200–800	As above.
Netball	30–60 mins 2–3 times weekly	200–600	Tones arms and lower body. Improves all-round strength and stamina.
Swimming	10–20 mins 2–3 times weekly	400–800	Excellent keep-fit sport, improves all-round strength, stamina and suppleness.
Running/ jogging	10–20 mins 2–3 times weekly	200–800	Benefits leg muscles, boosts stamina and the cardiovascular system.

RECREATION AND RELAXATION

Dancing	20–30 mins 2–3 times weekly	200–700	Eases tension, improves fitness, suppleness, co-ordination and stamina.
Martial arts	30–60 mins twice a week	400–1000	Improves strength, co-ordination, reflexes and stamina.
Yoga	30–60 mins 2–3 times weekly	125–175	Improves posture and suppleness. Soothes muscular and mental tension.
Golf	60–120 mins 2–3 times weekly	250–550	Improves flexibility, stamina and co-ordination.

TEN-MINUTE TIP

It's your move!

Experts recommend we raise our heart rate for 20 minutes three times a week to improve and maintain fitness levels. If you do any of the following exercises for ten minutes each day, you'll more than meet your weekly vitality quota.

- Power walking
- Cycling
- Rebounding
- Skipping
- Stairwalking
- Swimming

CHAPTER 10

Relaxation
Taking the strain
out of your face

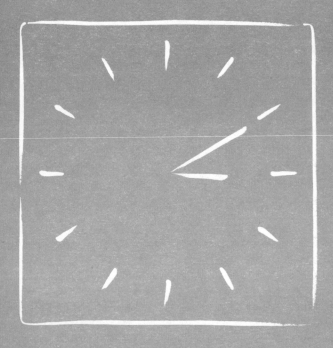

Stress eats away at your health, your looks and your vitality. Long term, it increases both the risk of illness and premature ageing. Lines, poor skin tone, lacklustre hair and persistent skin and scalp conditions are all triggered by chronic tension. It's small wonder, then, that when you're over-stressed your confidence suffers too. Taking time out to relax is a vital step to feeling great about yourself.

Early man had a hard time just staying alive, but he knew how to tackle life's knocks head-on. His response was simple and direct – either club it or leg it. Our sophisticated, 'buttoned up' attitude to pressure may not be a personal best on the evolution scale. Basically, we're still geared to what psychologists call the 'fight or flight' response, but we do everything in our power to suppress what's only natural.

Bottling up stress, say doctors and psychologists, is the underlying cause of at least 50 per cent of all physical and mental problems including depression, heart disease, some skin diseases and allergies such as asthma. Stress is also implicated in cancer, some forms of diabetes, colitis and irritable bowel syndrome. It overloads the immune system and diverts energy away from the body's natural healing and maintenance processes, and studies show that people under stress are far more likely to succumb to infections and less likely to recover quickly.

Stress is also a major factor of premature ageing which inhibits cell regeneration and instead generates free radical activity. Our skin is bound to suffer – worry lines become etched on our face and we look pinched, drawn and weary. Our body language says we're defensive, even defeated. Head down and shoulders hunched, we do not exactly radiate vitality. Worse, the physical clenching of stressed muscles inhibits circulation, limits mobility and may establish degenerative diseases.

Physical pain and feeling overwhelmed by pressure may force us into negative patterns such as drinking too much alcohol, oversleeping, overeating or overworking. Our poor self-esteem can isolate us from family and friends and this deepens our depression. But at the end of the day, only we can solve our problems. We owe it to ourselves to start, by finally busting stress and boosting our appetite for life.

WHAT HAPPENS WHEN YOU'RE STRESSED?

The fight or flight response is a complex chemical chain reaction which affects the entire body. Amazingly, the whole process takes nano-seconds. Say you suffer a shock. First, your senses become heightened as the threat looms. Then your brain assesses information received and prepares the body for action. Hormones flood the system and electrical impulses shoot through both the conscious system which is controlled by willpower and the autonomic system which, independent of will, controls the organs and regulates bodily functions. The hypothalamus – the brain's most primitive centre – triggers the production of three main stress hormones: adrenaline (or epinephrine), produced by the adrenal glands just above the kidneys, raises the heartbeat, blood pressure, breathing rate and blood sugar levels, so the body is energized; cortisol, also produced in the adrenal glands, increases the blood clotting rate and energizes the organs by converting stored fat into glucose. At the same time, the brain itself produces endorphins – neurochemicals that kill pain and produce that famous euphoric high.

> *For wellbeing's sake, we should get on top of stress before it overwhelms us*

Now you're all wired up, what's your next move? Convention makes it difficult to run or punch your way out, or even to burst into hot angry tears. In our superhuman effort to pull ourselves together, we're blocking an important physical and emotional release. In time, our system can dump a certain amount of the build-up and we calm down. But if the stress is sustained or repeated over long periods, our self-defence mechanism turns inwards and self-destruction begins. For wellbeing's sake, we should get on top of stress before it overwhelms us.

SIX STEPS TO BEAT STRESS

- **Don't bottle it up.** Discuss your problems with your partner or close friend. They may help you to see your problem more clearly. Recognize when you need to seek professional help. This isn't a sign of weakness, but a determination to exert your own power over the situation.
- **Laugh at it.** Laughter is a fabulous healer that takes the sting out of difficult situations and diffuses anger on the spot. It also boosts oxygen and endorphins – the body's feelgood chemicals.
- **Cry about it.** Tears have been found to contain stress

chemicals, proving that you really can – and should – sob stress out of your system. Some experts say that if men learned to cry more, they could cut the risk of heart disease.

- **Exercise.** Burn off stress-generated energy before it burns you up. A study at the University of British Columbia in Vancouver shows that 20–30 minutes of aerobic exercise which raises your heart rate to about 120 beats per minute at least three times a week can lower depression and anxiety within 12 weeks.

- **Manage it.** Tell yourself you can cope. Then get organized. Tackle important issues early to get them off your mind. Make space for them by not taking on anything trivial. Doing one thing well is more satisfying than trying to juggle several.

- **Give yourself TLC.** Treat yourself to something delicious. Pamper yourself in an aromatherapy bath or book a facial or massage. Do something you love, such as reading, dancing or watching a feelgood video. Then congratulate yourself. You've earned it.

BREATHING THE STRESS RIGHT OUT OF YOUR CELLS

Breathing is fundamental to relaxation. We breathe instinctively, but most of us use only around half our lung capacity. Sadly, a sexily heaving bodice is an obvious stress symptom that means oxygen is reaching the upper lungs only. Our cells need a good supply of oxygen in order to carry out their biochemical functions. In beauty terms, oxygen contributes to that fresh, youthful-looking radiance that gives healthy skin its glow. Shallow breathing means that the air sacs in our lungs absorb too little oxygen, leaving excess carbon dioxide in the tissues to be recirculated by the bloodstream. During stress or panic attacks, rapid, extremely shallow breaths cause hyperventilation – too little oxygen goes in and too much carbon dioxide goes out. The lungs respond by shutting down until oxygen levels normalize. The resulting feeling of tightness increases the panic. Inhaling into your own cupped hands or a paper bag for a couple of minutes regulates your air balance by forcing you to reinhale carbon diox-

> *A sexily heaving bodice is an obvious stress symptom*

ide. However, it's best to prevent a panic attack in the first place, and the way to do this is by learning breath control.

- Lie on a bed or on the floor. Rest both your hands just below your ribs, fingertips almost touching.
- Breathe through your nostrils. Inhale deeply so that you feel your ribs expanding and your stomach rising. Your fingertips should also move up and apart.
- Hold the breath for a count of five.
- Breathe out all the air smoothly. Feel your ribs collapse down and in, your stomach sink back and your fingertips almost touch.
- Repeat three or four times, then relax and breathe naturally. Then start the sequence again. If you start to feel dizzy, relax and breathe naturally.

Try not to do this exercise in polluted atmospheres, such as with the window open to a busy main road. Remember car exhaust fumes expel carbon dioxide and generate free radicals. To combat this, ionizers emit beneficial, negatively charged ions such as are found in sea or mountain air. These have the ability to 'ground' dust, smoke and pollution particles and are particularly recommended for asthma sufferers. Negative ions also boost alertness, reduce aggression and promote positive moods. Use ionizers at home and in the office.

MEDITATION TO EASE YOUR MIND

Meditation gives your mind time out from stress. This ancient Eastern technique has proven medical benefits, including lowering blood pressure and reducing the risk of heart disease. Our minds are constantly bombarded with information, whether we're conscious of it or not. Watching TV may seem relaxing, but your mind still has to process data. Meditation prevents information overload by focusing the mind on a single, simple thing. There are several methods you can use. Begin each by finding a comfortable position and make sure you will be able to stay warm and quiet for at least 20 minutes. Start with deep breathing (see above) until your body begins to relax.

- Breath meditation is a simple technique you can use anywhere. Empty your mind of everything, except your breathing. Focus on your breath as it comes in and goes out. Allow yourself to feel your ribs and stomach rising and falling. If you have trouble concentrating, try counting your breaths in sequences of ten.
- Mantra meditation is the method taught in Transcendental Meditation (TM). A mantra is a personal secret word with no intellectual meaning, usually given to you by a teacher. Alternatively, meditate to the classic sound 'Om' (pronounced 'aum'), the Eastern word said to embody universal love. Repeat it slowly and steadily in time to your breathing, concentrating on its pure sound. If conscious thoughts float into your mind, don't try to block them. Instead, actively acknowledge them, then breathe them out and focus on your mantra again.
- Object meditation focuses on a

Meditation gives your mind time out from stress

small object instead of a word. Use a candle, crystal or stone which is easy to carry around. Place it a few feet away from you at eye level or just below to prevent tiring your eye muscles. Concentrate on the object's shape, texture, even smell, and sense its weight and energy.

YOGA TO STRETCH AWAY STRESS

Yoga benefits everyone, whatever their age. Central to Ayurveda, India's ancient natural medicine, yoga is now hugely popular in the West as a successful method of relaxing and balancing the mind, body and spirit. The asanas, or postures, are a series of gentle stretches which promote balance, flexibility, strength and muscle control throughout the entire body. Even the internal organs are 'massaged' by special movements. There are various schools of yoga now in the West, some more dynamic than others. Whichever you choose, the rules are basically the same. Always go at your own pace and never force a posture. If it hurts, stop. The best way to learn yoga is from a qualified teacher who will gently guide you. Meanwhile, practise this relaxing technique whenever you have a spare half hour, or before bed to help you get off to sound sleep.

- Lie down in a quiet, dark room. Place a pillow or cushion under your head and knees to take the strain off your spine. Cover yourself with a blanket to keep warm. Let your arms rest loosely at your sides.
- Take a couple of deep breaths as you relax, sighing out the tension. Take your time to do this, enjoying the luxury.
- When you're ready, starting with your toes and travelling upwards to the face and scalp, consciously tell every inch of your body to relax. If this is difficult, try tensing the area then relaxing it to experience full stress-release.
- Relax your face. Yawn, opening your mouth widely. Purse

your lips tightly, then blow air through them as you relax. Frown like you mean it, then release the emotion. Raise the eyebrows to shift the scalp and let go. Screw up your entire face – mouth, nose, cheeks, eyelids, brow – then relax.

- When your whole body is relaxed, concentrate on that warm, heavy feeling. Breathe rhythmically, telling yourself you feel more relaxed with each breath.
- Stay that way for around 15 minutes. Then gently come to by stretching and moving your limbs until you feel ready to get up and go again.

T'AI CHI: REPLACING TENSION WITH GRACE

T'ai Chi Chuan is an ancient Chinese technique combining philosophy with movement. Practised by millions of Chinese daily, this 'meditation in motion' encourages the balance of negative yin and positive yang energies so that chi, or life force, flows smoothly. A series of postures and breathing techniques are performed slowly in a balletic sequence to improve muscle control and body–mind harmony. They're not strenuous, as their aim is to promote grace, tranquillity and optimum use of your energy. Ideally, you should practise T'ai Chi in the open air, on grass and first thing in the morning to set you up for the day, but you can try this loosen-up, warm-up technique any time, especially before an energy-intensive event.

- Stand with your feet still and slightly wider than your hips. Swing your arms slowly from side to side, keeping your shoulders level, but turning your body as you go. Clear your mind and concentrate on smooth, flowing movements.
- Now, as you swing your arms, deepen your swing by letting each foot in turn turn out to the side in the direction of your arms.

- Finally, raise your arms slowly above your head, elbows relaxed and hands slightly apart. Move both arms together to trace a wide circle as you bend your body to the side, down to the floor and up to the ceiling again.

CONVINCE YOURSELF YOU'RE CALM

Can you will yourself to be calmer? Use your imagination. In hospitals, positive visualization is encouraged to help fight disease, including cancer. Patients are urged to imagine their tumour being bombarded by infection-fighting cells, like a *Star Wars*-style video game. Researchers say aggressive visualization improves recovery chances. You can soothe yourself better too by visualizing a tranquil scenario.

- Make sure you feel warm, safe and comfortable.
- Play gentle, quiet music or sounds from nature such as the sea or rain.
- Burn a relaxing oil or aromatherapy candle – camomile, lavender and neroli all work well.
- Use positive affirmations to tell yourself 'I am safe, at peace with myself and relaxed.'
- Imagine you're somewhere tranquil – a place where you've been happy or relaxed, or an imaginary desert island or secret garden.
- Imagine the warm sun on your body as you let colours, sounds and scents flood your mind's eye and wash gently over you.
- As you become expert, you can 'switch off' and allow new images to automatically come into your mind. This can often bring new insight and put a fresh perspective on old problems. But remember, if you don't enjoy what you see,

you can always change the channel by simply changing your mind.

Using stress

Stress can be good for us. Eustress, or 'healthy stress', is the kick behind clear, creative thinking and achieving personal goals. Without the occasional rush of adrenaline, we'd be too laid-back for our own good. But while eustress can be euphoric, too much of a good thing can turn to jittery hyper-activity. Come down naturally from a 'high' without crashing. Exercise it out of your system or use a relaxation technique until you feel satisfyingly tired.

TEN-MINUTE TIP

Calm down!

This easy exercise is based on autogenics, a simple form of self-hypnosis. Stressed executives, airline pilots, even astronauts have successfully used this technique since its introduction by German psychiatrist Johannes Schults in the 1930s. Go for it any time, anywhere – in traffic jams or trains, before meetings or in bed. Practise it each day, and the stress-release response becomes automatic.

- Lie down or sit comfortably. Repeat these commands to yourself slowly and quietly, visualizing each part of the body in turn. Do this over and over until you feel yourself relaxing.
- My arms and legs are heavy and warm.
- My heartbeat is calm and regular.
- My forehead is cool and clear.
- My neck and shoulders are heavy.
- I am at peace.

BIBLIOGRAPHY

Alexander, Jane, *Supertherapies*. Bantam Books, London.

Bentley, Vicci, *Forever Young*. Carlton Books, London.

Brown, Bobbi & Iverson, Annemarie, *Bobbi Brown Beauty*. Ebury Press, London.

Burke, Karen, *Great Skin for Life*. Hamlyn, London.

Burke, Karen, *Thin Thighs for Life*. Hamlyn, London.

Gross, Kim Johnson et al, *Woman's Face*. Knopf.

Hillman, Carolynn, *Love Your Looks*. Simon & Schuster.

Hutton, Deborah, *Vogue Futures*. Condé Nast Books.

Kingsley, Philip, *Hair, an Owner's Handbook*. Aurum Press, London.

Maggio, Carole, *Facercise*. Boxtree, London.

Maxwell-Hudson, Clare, *The Complete Book of Massage*. Dorling Kindersley, London.

Mindell, Earl, *The Anti-Ageing Bible*. Souvenir Press, London.

Sutcliffe, Jenny, *Relaxation Techniques*. Headline, London.

Woodham, Anne, *HEA Guide to Complementary Medicine and Therapies*. HEA, London.

also available from
THE ORION PUBLISHING GROUP

☐ **Apples & Pears** £3.99
GLORIA THOMAS
0 75281 604 7

☐ **Are You Getting Enough?**
£4.99
ANGELA DOWDEN
0 75281 702 7

☐ **Arousing Aromas** £3.99
KAY COOPER
0 75281 546 6

☐ **Body Foods For Women**
£6.99
JANE CLARKE
0 75280 922 9

☐ **Coping With Your Premature Baby** £4.99
DR PENNY STANWAY
0 75281 596 2

☐ **Cranks Light** £6.99
NADINE ABENSUR
0 75283 727 3

☐ **Cranks Recipe Book** £6.99
CRANKS RESTAURANTS
1 85797 140 X

☐ **Eat Safely** £3.99
JANET WRIGHT
0 75281 544 X

☐ **First Baby After Thirty ... or Forty?** £4.99
DR PENNY STANWAY
0 75281 595 4

☐ **The Good Mood Guide**
£4.99
ROS & JEREMY HOLMES
0 75282 584 4

☐ **Harmonise Your Home**
£4.99
GRAHAM GUNN
0 75281 665 9

☐ **Health Spa at Home** £3.99
JOSEPHINE FAIRLEY
0 75281 545 8

☐ **Juice Up Your Energy Levels**
£3.99
LESLEY WATERS
0 75281 602 0

☐ **Miscarriage: What Every Woman Needs to Know**
£7.99
PROFESSOR LESLEY REGAN
0 75283 757 5

☐ **Natural Painkillers** £4.99
NIKKI BRADFORD
0 75281 603 9

☐ **The New Cranks Recipe Book** £6.99
NADINE ABENSUR
0 75281 677 2

☐ **No Fuss Fat Loss** £4.99
MAGGIE DRUMMOND
0 75283 724 9

☐ **Sensitive Skin** £4.99
JOSEPHINE FAIRLEY
0 75281 547 4

☐ **Spring Clean Your System**
£3.99
JANE GARTON
0 75281 601 2

☐ **Vegetarian Slimming** £6.99
ROSE ELLIOT
0 75280 173 2

All Orion/Phoenix/Indigo titles are available at your local bookshop or from the following address:

Mail Order Department
Littlehampton Book Services
FREEPOST BR535
Worthing, West Sussex, BN13 3BR
telephone 01903 828503, *facsimile* 01903 828802
e-mail MailOrders@lbsltd.co.uk
(Please ensure that you include full postal address details)

Payment can be made either by credit/debit card (Visa, Mastercard, Access and Switch accepted) or by sending a £ Sterling cheque or postal order made payable to *Littlehampton Book Services*.
DO NOT SEND CASH OR CURRENCY.

Please add the following to cover postage and packing

UK and BFPO:
£1.50 for the first book, and 50p for each additional book to a maximum of £3.50

Overseas and Eire:
£2.50 for the first book plus £1.00 for the second book and 50p for each additional book ordered

---

BLOCK CAPITALS PLEASE

name of cardholder ....

....

address of cardholder ....

....

....

....

postcode ....

delivery address
(if different from cardholder)

....

....

....

....

postcode ....

☐ I enclose my remittance for £.............................

☐ please debit my Mastercard/Visa/Access/Switch (delete as appropriate)

card number ☐☐☐☐☐☐☐☐☐☐☐☐☐☐☐☐

expiry date ☐☐☐☐   Switch issue no. ☐☐

signature ....

prices and availability are subject to change without notice